MW01118630

GETTING READY FOR

BABY

The Ultimate Organizer for the Mom-to-Be

by Hélène Tragos Stelian

CHRONICLE BOOKS

SAN FRANCISCO

Copyright © 2001 by Hélène Tragos Stelian. Illustrations © 2001 by Anders Wenngren for Art Department. All rights reserved. No part of this book may be reproduced in any form, except for personal use, without written permission from the publisher.

Library of Congress Cataloging-in-Publication Data
Stelian, Hélène Tragos.
    Getting ready for baby : the ultimate organizer for the mom-to-be / by Hélène Tragos Stelian.
        p. cm.
    Includes bibliographical references.
    ISBN 978-0-8118-2941-0
    1. Mothers—Life skills guides. 2. Pregnant women—Life skills guides. 3. Pregnancy—Popular works.
    4. Childbirth—Popular works. 5. Infants—Health and hygiene. 6. Infants' supplies. I. Title

    HQ759 .S686 2001
    306.874'3—dc21   2001028798

Printed in Hong Kong   Design by Alethea Morrison
Typeset in Futura and Filosofia   Illustrations by Anders Wenngren for Art Department

Chronicle Books LLC
680 Second Street
San Francisco, CA 94107
www.chroniclebooks.com

ISBN 978-0-8118-2941-0   10

The information contained in this journal is meant to be taken as advice only, and to supplement but not replace the guidance of a medical doctor. Consult your physician for questions relating to your pregnancy, your health, and the health of your newborn.

ACKNOWLEDGMENTS

Grateful thanks go to many new and seasoned mothers for their "Real Mom Tips", feedback, and enthusiastic support of this project: Ann Airey, Diana Aixalá, Catherine Briggs, Jetta Bushonville, Becky Chodes, Jeannine Everett, Barbara Golub, Kate Hansell, Caroline Heming, Anita Khosla, Sharon Komlofske, Marcie Prokupek, Helen Shayne, and Amalia Stachowiak, not to mention numerous moms who lent advice on a more informal basis.

I am also indebted to the following individuals for their expert contributions to this book: Holly Casele, M.D.; Karen S. Gillett, R.N., B.S.N.; William Grobman, M.D.; David W. Nichols, M.D.; Dawn Pepsnik, R.N.C.; Andrew Roth, M.D.; Philip Shayne, M.D.; Nicolae Schon, M.D.; Celeste Sheppard, M.D.; Lori Weiss, M.D.; Terri Brax, Owner, Teacher Care; Mary Jane Sellers, President, American Registry for Nannies & Sitters; Ruth Taxy, Director, Glencoe Junior Kindergarten.

Several writers provided much-needed direction, critique, contacts, and encouragement: Kathy McDonald, Anne Miano, and Debbie Seaman. In addition, my sister, Katherine Tragos, did the initial book design and illustration, which were critical to the acceptance of my book proposal.

I'd like to recognize the babysitters who took such loving and patient care of our daughters, allowing me the time to devote to this project: Iania Santana, Pam Girard, and Missy Kuhman Smith.

This book could not have come to light without my agent, Jeanne Fredericks, who believed in it from the start and helped me navigate the publishing waters. Many thanks go to Chronicle Books for sharing my vision and for bringing it to life. I am especially grateful to Debra Lande for recognizing my book's potential and to Carey Jones for her insightful edits.

Finally, I cannot express the depth of my love and gratitude for my husband Peter Stelian, who allowed me the freedom and the opportunity to pursue my dream, and became my greatest cheerleader. I could not wish for a more wonderful partner.

TO MY SILLY MONKEYS,

BIANCA AND INDIGO

CONTENTS

HEALTHCARE FOR BABY

CHILDCARE

RESOURCES

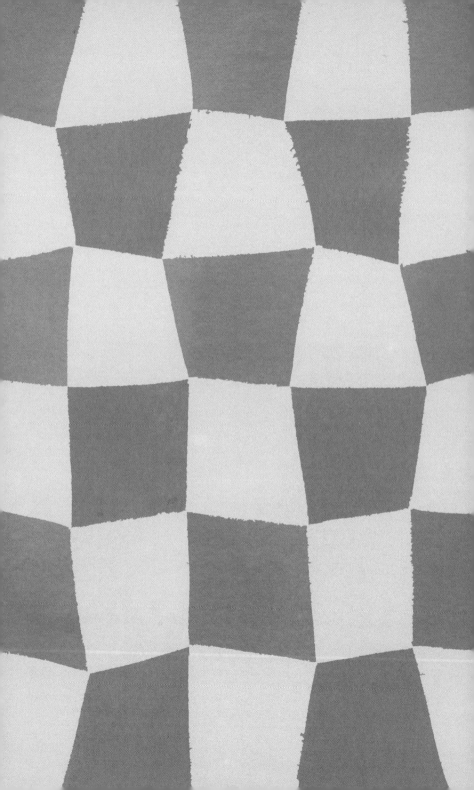

INTRODUCTION

Dear mom-to-be,

Congratulations on your pregnancy!

When I found out I was pregnant with twins, I felt both elated and anxious. On the one hand, I pictured cozy family moments with smiling babies; I couldn't believe we'd have to wait nine months to meet our girls. On the other hand, I realized we had no clue how to raise a child, let alone two; nine months would never be enough time to get ready.

Of course, one can never be "ready." In fact, I'm learning as I go along. Having children has challenged every aspect of my life, led me to reexamine my priorities, and redefined my goals. My world has changed permanently, and I'm delighted. My daughters remind me every day of the power of love, the wonder of nature, the responsibilities of parenting, and the pleasure of silliness.

Your journey into motherhood is just beginning; it will be a long, intensely personal expedition. I won't pretend to guide you over its soaring peaks and challenging valleys. My wish is to help you sort through the more practical aspects of welcoming a new baby, from shopping for a newborn layette to packing your hospital bag, finding the perfect pediatrician to setting up your nursery. Ultimately, I'd like to make preparing for your baby as easy and stress-free as possible so you can focus on enjoying your pregnancy and bonding with your newborn...in other words, on beginning your journey.

Ready to take the plunge? Skim through this book to get an overall sense of the road ahead, how this planner can help, and the tremendous resources at your disposal. Then, turn to the THINGS TO DO chapter and get started! Remember to customize this planner as you go along: Add your own notes and to do's, complete the charts and checklists, and run multiple copies of the questionnaires and logs. In short, do anything that makes this book work harder for you. And always keep it nearby so you'll have key information right at your fingertips.

I wish you a peaceful pregnancy, a healthy baby, and a delightful passage into motherhood.

Hélène

KEY CONTACTS

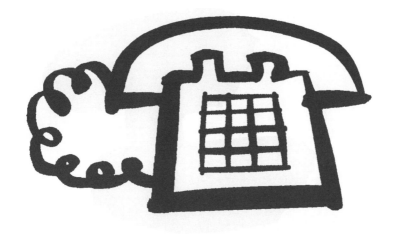

● ◦ ◦ **BASICS**

NAME

ADDRESS

EXPECTED DATE
OF DELIVERY

HOME PHONE   HOME FAX

WORK PHONE   WORK FAX

CELL PHONE   PAGER

NAME

HOME PHONE   WORK PHONE

CELL PHONE   PAGER

OTHER INFO

ALTERNATE LABOR COACH NAME AND PHONE

TAXI COMPANY NAME AND PHONE

INSURANCE NAME   **PHONE**

OB NAME   **PHONE**

OTHER DOCTORS

INSURANCE NAME   **PHONE**

PEDIATRICIAN NAME   **PHONE**

OTHER DOCTORS

PHARMACY NAME   **PHONE**

PHARMACY ADDRESS

HOSPITAL NAME   **PHONE**

HOSPITAL ADDRESS

DIRECTIONS/PARKING

FREQUENTLY CALLED NUMBERS

NAME	PHONE

THINGS TO DO

● ● ● REAL MOM TIPS: GETTING IT ALL DONE

Once you're past the initial excitement of being pregnant, you may feel overwhelmed by the number of issues to consider and the many items you need to purchase. Family and friends may ask: Will you have an amnio? Do you want to know the sex of the baby? Did you sign up for a childbirth class yet? Do you favor an epidural? Have you chosen a pediatrician? Would you have your boy circumcised? Have you written wills? What will you name your baby? Wait a second...time out!

Maintain your sanity, thanks to the following advice from recent new moms.

TAKE IT EASY

Unless you've just learned you're 6 months pregnant, you can afford to take it easy. The first trimester, focus on taking care of yourself, whether that means getting extra sleep or experimenting with nausea-reducing snacks. As you become more accustomed to being pregnant, talk to other moms, start reading a few maternity books, and discuss matters of immediate concern with your partner.

TAKE ONE STEP AT A TIME

The checklists that follow are meant to cover most to do's in a pregnancy and are organized in order of importance, by trimester. Add your own personal tasks in the blank spaces provided. Once you have a game plan, it will be easier to relax and get things done as needed instead of worrying about what you're forgetting. Don't stress yourself out by cramming all your to do's into the first trimester, but don't procrastinate until the last month either: You never know when a baby will make an early appearance.

ASK FOR HELP

Family and friends will want to help, so go ahead and ask, whether for a shoulder to lean on when you're anxious or for help shopping for a car seat. Other women often enjoy sharing their own experiences and advice; you'll be surprised at how soon you'll be returning the favor for other moms-to-be.

● ● ● **TO-DO CHECKLIST**

Here's a list of things to remember throughout your pregnancy and in the first months after your baby's birth. Add everything you'd like to accomplish during each trimester and check off when tasks are completed.

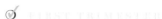

- Understand your health insurance plan, including what services will and will not be covered.

- Interview and choose your obstetrician and the hospital where you'll deliver. Fill out the OB Basics form (in the HEALTHCARE FOR MOM chapter).

- Meet with your OB. Come prepared with your Health History form as well as your list of questions. Keep track of the doctor's instructions with the OB Visits/Calls forms (in the HEALTHCARE FOR MOM chapter).

- Make changes to your diet and exercise habits as directed by your OB. Consider signing up for special pregnancy classes such as yoga or water aerobics.

- Decide, with your OB's help, if you want prenatal testing such as an amnio or CVS and schedule the testing.

- Understand your employer's maternity leave policy.

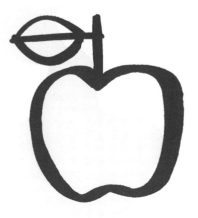

- Start saving for the extra expenses of a new baby. Track how much you spend so you're sure to stick to your budget.

- Keep track of insurance submissions, payments, and calls (see the HEALTHCARE FOR MOM chapter).

- Purchase or borrow a few pregnancy books and start reading (see the RESOURCES chapter for suggestions).

- Collect pediatrician and childcare recommendations (see the HEALTHCARE FOR BABY and CHILDCARE chapters).

- If you plan on hiring a baby nurse to help with your newborn, call friends and neighbors for leads. Line up a nurse now because they often get booked months in advance.

- Visit your dentist to make sure you take proper care of your teeth and gums, which are more vulnerable during pregnancy.

- _____

- _____

- _____

SECOND TRIMESTER

- Ask to borrow maternity and baby items from family and friends; keep track with the Borrowed Items logs (in the SHOPPING FOR MOM and SHOPPING FOR BABY chapters).

- Purchase maternity clothing as needed (see checklists in the SHOPPING FOR MOM chapter, catalogs and books in the RESOURCES chapter, and maternity stores in your phone book).

- Purchase or borrow parenting, baby care, and baby name books (see the RESOURCES chapter).

○ Inform your place of work about your pregnancy (as needed).

○ Enroll in childbirth, infant CPR/First Aid, breastfeeding, childcare, and other classes at your hospital of choice.

○ Decide if you wish to hire a doula (a trained coach who will help you through labor and delivery); if so, look in the RESOURCES chapter, gather recommendations, and plan interviews now.

○ Decide on nursery colors and theme and start laying out your baby's room (see the Nursery Plan-o-gram in the SHOPPING FOR BABY chapter).

○ Research and order/buy major baby items (see checklists in the SHOPPING FOR BABY chapter, catalogs and books in the RESOURCES chapter, and baby stores in your phone book).

○ Determine your long-term childcare needs and begin researching options. If you are leaning toward using a daycare or hiring an *au pair,* make appropriate phone calls now (see the CHILDCARE and RESOURCES chapters).

○ Think through who will care for older siblings and household pets when delivery day arrives, and make sure your game plan covers labor beginning in the middle of the night or when your labor coach is away.

○ Sign up an older sibling for a tour and new sibling class at your hospital. Purchase some children's books about becoming a big brother or sister and make a big deal out of this new role. Include siblings in baby preparations.

○ Begin taking monthly "belly pictures" as a visual reminder of your pregnancy.

○ ....

○ ....

○ ....

○ ....

( ) Get a pager for your partner or labor coach to carry.

( ) Pre-register at the hospital and become familiar with parking, directions to the labor and delivery floor, etc.

( ) Finalize health insurance plans for your baby.

( ) Interview and choose a pediatrician and fill out the Pediatrician Basics chart (in the HEALTHCARE FOR BABY chapter).

( ) Decide whether you would circumcise if you have a baby boy.

( ) Continue to read books on parenting and baby care.

( ) Write or update your wills and consider life insurance.

( ) Decide on your baby's name (see books in the RESOURCES chapter).

( ) Decorate the nursery early on so any paint or new carpet fumes have a chance to dissipate before baby's arrival. It's also best not to have the mom-to-be or other children inhale these fumes, so ventilate the area well.

( ) Finalize sibling and pet care for when you go into labor, as well as baby nurse help (if using) for after the birth.

( ) Research childcare, based on your needs. If you're planning to use an agency to find a nanny, sign up and fill out required forms now (see the CHILDCARE and RESOURCES chapters).

( ) Purchase smaller items for your baby (see the SHOPPING FOR BABY chapter).

( ) Sign up with a diaper service if choosing cloth diapers.

( ) Purchase nursing items and clothing (see the SHOPPING FOR MOM and RESOURCES chapters).

( ) Finalize details of your maternity leave with your employer.

Decide on birth announcements and thank-you cards. Pre-address and stamp announcement envelopes; ask to get the envelopes early if ordering custom announcements (see the BACK HOME and RESOURCES chapters).

Write thank-you notes for baby shower or other gifts. Keep track with the Gifts and Thank-You's log (in the BABY SHOWER AND GIFTS chapter).

Fill out the Emergency Information chart (in the HEALTHCARE FOR BABY chapter) and post it by all telephones.

Start baby-proofing your home and study dos and don'ts (see the Baby-Proofing Checklist later in this chapter).

Purchase a gift from the new baby to his/her older sibling and let the older sibling choose a gift for the new baby.

Begin dropping hints now if you're expecting a gift from your partner after the delivery. Many people are not aware of this custom.

○

○

○

Pack your hospital bag (see the LABOR AND DELIVERY chapter).

Fill out your Birthing Plan (in the LABOR AND DELIVERY chapter) and discuss it with your OB at your next appointment.

Write your prioritized list of people to call from the hospital (see the LABOR AND DELIVERY chapter). Consider buying a prepaid phone card if a phone will not be readily available after the delivery or if you'll be making long-distance calls. Find out your hospital's policy on cell phone use.

- Install your car seat securely (see safety organizations and Web sites for tips, in the RESOURCES chapter).

- Run through the LABOR AND DELIVERY chapter with your labor coach to make sure he/she understands all the responsibilities as well as your preferences before delivery day.

- Prewash all baby clothing and linens.

- Arrange and organize all your baby items in the nursery and kitchen. Sterilize baby bottles and nipples in boiling water.

- Reserve a rental breast pump or purchase one, including all necessary attachments (unless your hospital will provide them).

- Stock up on household basics.

- Cook and freeze prepared meals. Make a list of carryout and delivery places for after the birth.

- Get recommendations for mother and child classes so you're ready to enroll when the time comes.

- Plan for a religious ceremony or other celebration (see the BACK HOME chapter).

- _____

- _____

- _____

AFTER THE BIRTH

- Call your health insurance company to inform them of baby's name and arrival.

- Get a social security number for your baby, ideally through the hospital to save you a call later.

- Call in birth announcement information if you're having them printed (see the Custom Announcements in the BACK HOME chapter).

- If you're including photos in your birth announcement mailing, take a picture of your newborn and have it copied.

- Send out birth announcements (see the Announcement Mailing List in the BACK HOME chapter).

- Send a thank-you note or gift basket to helpful hospital staff if you did not get to it before leaving the hospital.

- Have your partner pick up your rental breast pump and any last-minute items you need.

- Keep track of your baby's breast milk or formula intake as well as wet/soiled diapers with the Feeding and Diapering log (in the BACK HOME chapter).

- Keep track of baby gifts and good deeds with the Gifts and Thank-You's log (see the BABY SHOWER AND GIFTS chapter).

- Send out thank-you notes as your time and energy allow but try not to let the list grow so long that it becomes overwhelming.

- Make your two-week pediatrician appointment. Plan to bring your Health History (in the HEALTHCARE FOR MOM chapter), your Feeding and Diapering log (in the HEALTHCARE FOR BABY chapter), and a list of questions. Note baby's medical information on the forms in the HEALTHCARE FOR BABY chapter.

- Keep track of insurance submissions, payments, and calls (see the HEALTHCARE FOR MOM and HEALTHCARE FOR BABY chapters).

- Make your six-week obstetrician appointment.

- Finalize plans for a religious or other celebration (see the BACK HOME chapter).

- Interview for childcare, if you'll need it after your baby is born (see the CHILDCARE chapter).

Make changes to your federal tax exemptions to include your baby (change your W-4 with your employer to claim a dependent). Take advantage of child tax credits, as well as childcare credits or dependent-care flexible spending accounts.

Wash or dry-clean borrowed maternity clothing and return items to their owners with a note of thanks and a small gift (refer back to your Borrowed Items log in the SHOPPING FOR MOM chapter and see gift ideas in the BABY SHOWER AND GIFTS chapter).

Fill out the Medical Treatment Authorization form and post it along with the Emergency Information and Baby's Health charts prior to leaving your baby in someone else's care (see the HEALTHCARE FOR BABY chapter).

Receive a free signed congratulatory note from the President. Send the baby's name, address, and birth date to: White House Greetings Office, Room 39, Washington, DC 20500.

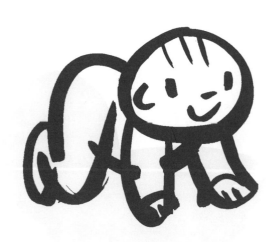

● ● ● BABY-PROOFING CHECKLIST

*It's only a matter of months before your baby will begin exploring your
home. Why not get an early start on childproofing? Get down on
your hands and knees so you can see potential dangers from a child's
perspective. Get the supplies you'll need at your local hardware or baby
equipment store, or through safety catalogs and Web sites (see the*
RESOURCES *chapter). You can also look in the Yellow Pages for childproofing
experts in your area who can do the job for you.*

Make sure your home has working smoke/fire detectors on each floor,
including in the kitchen and garage and in/near each bedroom. (Test all
detectors monthly and replace batteries as needed, at least once a
year.) Keep fire extinguishers on each floor, including in the kitchen, and
know how to use them. Store a fire escape ladder within easy reach in
all occupied upper-level rooms; plan and practice an escape route every 6
months with family and caregivers.

Place carbon monoxide detectors on each level of your house, particularly
near fireplaces and garages, and in bedrooms.

Have working flashlights handy in the kitchen and your bedroom in the event
of a power failure.

Check all painted surfaces for lead and have all lead paint professionally
removed. Don't let baby play near deteriorating paint. Also check your home
for asbestos and have it removed professionally. (Look in the Yellow Pages
under lead and asbestos testing/removal.)

Set your water heater to 120°F or less.

Post the Emergency Information, Baby's Health, and Medical Treatment Authorization forms in plain view by each phone (see the HEALTHCARE FOR BABY chapter).

○ Take an Infant CPR/First Aid class before baby's arrival and regular refresher courses as recommended. Post the CPR chart in a central location in your home. Make sure every individual caring for your child is certified.

○ Keep a First Aid kit handy (see the SHOPPING FOR BABY chapter).

○ Store poisonous or toxic substances out of reach in cabinets locked with safety latches. Examples: Cleaning and laundry products, chemicals and bug sprays, toiletries and perfumes, cosmetics and nail products, alcohol and tobacco, medicines and vitamins, painting and gardening products, car maintenance fluids and mothballs, potpourri and houseplants, tools and glues, markers and lead pencils, pet food and litter.

○ Store hazards out of reach in cabinets locked with safety latches. Examples: Firearms and ammunition, lawnmowers and other heavy equipment, fishing gear and tools, matches and lighters, glassware and breakables, knives and scissors, razors and blades, staplers and staples, sewing supplies and sharp items, foil and paper clips, jewelry.

○ While you're on your hands and knees, conduct a thorough hunt for items small enough to be choking hazards. Store all small items out of reach, from buttons to batteries, peanuts to popcorn, balloons to plastic bags. (Choking hazards include anything that fits into a cardboard toilet-paper tube.)

○ Cover all electrical outlets with child-resistant covers. Replace frayed electrical cords and never put electrical cords under rugs. Unplug and store all electrical appliances out of reach and away from sinks, toilets, and bathtubs. Put barriers in front of fans, fireplaces, radiators, floor lamps, and space heaters. Avoid halogen lamps, which can cause burns. Keep all sources of heat away from flammables like drapes and papers.

○ Keep all blind, drapery, electrical, and phone cords out of a baby's reach with cord shorteners. Use cord tubing and power strip covers to control multiple cords and outlets.

- Move furniture away from windows and make sure all windows lock securely, or install quick-release window guards.

- Screw all shelves and dressers to the walls using furniture wall straps. Secure all elevated items that could fall and crush a child, like a TV set that rests on a stand. Make sure all chests and toy boxes have slam-proof hinges.

- Use door pinch guards or doorstops to keep doors from slamming onto tiny fingers. Place knob guards on the doors of rooms to be kept out of bounds. Always keep doors leading outside securely locked. Replace doorstops that have removable rubber tips with one-piece doorstops.

- Place pads around the edges of coffee tables, low counters, and fireplace hearths, and install corner guards on any sharp furniture corners.

- Remove the keys from fireplace gas starters and secure all other fireplace tools and accessories.

- Secure floor vents with screws and place nonskid pads under area rugs.

- Mount safety gates (with screws, not pressure-mounted) at the tops and bottoms of staircases.

- Install plastic mesh or Plexiglas sheets on railing banisters that are more than 3 inches apart, particularly for balconies, decks, and staircases.

- Place colorful decals on large glass windows and doors so children can spot the glass and will not try to run through it.

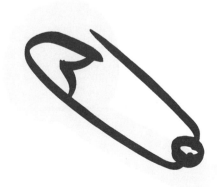

Remove all dry-cleaning bags from clothing immediately. Open up the ends of empty plastic bags and tie them up in knots before discarding them. Keep trash cans securely closed and out of reach.

Install non-slip bath mats, tub edge pads, and water faucet covers in the bathtub your baby will be using. Install toilet seat locks and remove toilet bowl cleaning inserts on all toilets. Keep toilet brushes and plungers out of baby's reach.

Install stove knob covers or a stove-front shield. Put safety straps on fridge, freezer, and oven doors. Install garbage disposal switch covers.

Make sure all your baby furniture and toys meet safety guidelines (see CPSC and JPMA in the RESOURCES chapter). Be especially vigilant with used items. Your crib should have no more than 2⅜ inches between slats and the mattress should fit snugly against all sides. Position your crib and changing table away from all cords, windows, heating vents, space heaters, and radiators. Make sure mobiles are securely installed and remove them once your baby can reach up and touch them. Lower the crib mattress when baby begins to sit and remove all bumper pads and toys (they can be used to climb out) when baby begins to stand. Stuffed animals should have embroidered eyes and features. Toys should not have removable small parts or long cords or ribbons.

Fence in your yard. Clean up all debris, mushrooms, animal feces, garbage and check for safety issues. Make sure any spas or pools are covered, fenced in, and secured with a lock, and that your automatic garage door has a mechanism that keeps the door from closing if it hits an obstacle. Keep your garage out of bounds to children. You may wish to hide a house key in a safe location outside the house in case you lock yourself out with your baby inside (while getting the mail, for example).

Make sure you've installed your car seat securely in the back seat of your car, facing to the rear, and get help if it moves more than 1 inch from side to side when you jiggle it (see safety Web sites, catalogs, and organizations in the RESOURCES chapter.)

DOS AND DON'TS

Always put your baby to sleep on his or her back, in fire-retardant sleepwear, on a firm mattress, and never put pillows or other soft bedding or toys in baby's crib (to reduce risk of Sudden Infant Death Syndrome—SIDS). Always raise the side railing when baby is in the crib.

Use only a cool-mist humidifier in baby's room (hot-mist ones can scald) and follow all maintenance instructions vigilantly.

Always throw out expired medications. Buy medicines, vitamins, and other hazardous substances with childproof caps whenever possible. Never refer to medicine or vitamins as candy.

Never leave a baby unattended on a bed or couch, on a high chair or changing table, in a bathtub or near water (from pools to toilets to buckets), outside or in a car, with a pet or young child, near stairs or active sources of heat (from ovens to space heaters), near dangerous substances or items, with food or a propped bottle.

Never hold a baby on your lap in the car; always strap a baby into the car seat.

Always use the safety straps on your car seat, bouncer seat, swing, changing table, and high chair. Never place a bouncer seat or car seat on an elevated surface.

Never handle hot/lit items (e.g. coffee, iron, cigarettes) near your baby or leave these items unattended.

Never use accordion-style gates or barriers, or walkers with wheels.

Use your stove's back burners and always turn pot handles toward the back of the stove. Always point knives and forks down in the dishwasher basket and keep the dishwasher door locked. Don't use tablecloths that can be pulled down (pulling plates and dinnerware onto your child). Make sure baby cups and dishware are made of unbreakable plastic or paper.

- Never leave a cord dangling from a table, desk, or counter.

- Always check the water temperature with your wrist or elbow before putting your baby in bathwater and empty the tub immediately after use.

- Teach your baby never to stand on furniture or in the tub.

- Keep your baby out of direct sunlight at all times, shield delicate skin with hats and long sleeves, and check with your pediatrician about the use of sunscreen and insect repellent.

- Remove loose threads, buttons and drawstrings from clothing, blankets, and toys. Never tie a pacifier or toy onto a string. Make sure baby clothing is not too tight at cuffs and collars.

- Stay on top of the latest product recalls: Parenting magazines and Web sites often publish big-name brand recalls (see the RESOURCES chapter) or you can have product recall information from the U.S. Consumer Product Safety Commission sent directly to your email address (register at www.cpsc.gov/about/subscribe.html).

- Always set a good example. Don't let your child see you standing on chairs, climbing over safety gates, or doing any of the things you're asking him/her not to do.

HEALTHCARE FOR MOM

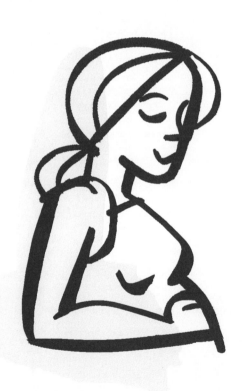

REAL MOM TIPS: PARTNERING WITH YOUR OBSTETRICIAN

Do you love your obstetrician? Do you look forward to visits? A great OB can help reduce pregnancy jitters and enhance the entire experience, particularly the first time around. It's vital that you're comfortable with your doctor's competence and approach, as well as with the other doctors in the practice.

Ask like-minded family, friends, co-workers, and other doctors for OB recommendations (note them in the Potential Obstetricians form), speak to the office staff to make sure your basic requirements are met (see below), then ask to interview the doctor, ideally in person and at least over the phone (see OB Interview form). In any case, visit the office before joining to assess its location, cleanliness, and atmosphere.

Consider these issues when choosing an OB.

BASIC REQUIREMENTS

Call the office and speak to a staff person in charge. Make sure the following basics meet your needs before requesting an interview with the OB.

1   **Insurance:** Is the practice covered by your insurance plan and accepting new patients? Will the staff process claims directly with your insurance company? Does the practice require a deposit for a portion of the estimated obstetrical costs?

2   **Certification and affiliation:** Are doctors in the practice board-certified by the American Board of Obstetrics and Gynecology, state-licensed, and affiliated with a reputable hospital? Tour the hospital to determine the following: Does it offer 24-hour in-house anesthesia and pediatric care? How well equipped is it to handle unexpected complications with you or your baby? (If you're at high risk for delivering a premature baby, you'll want a level III neonatal intensive care unit.) What security procedures are in place to protect babies in the nursery? How supportive is it regarding issues of

importance to you, whether nursing, using a doula, or rooming in with your baby? What programs and services does the hospital offer to new and expectant parents?

3 **Location and hours:** Is the office conveniently located near your home and/ or work? You'll be seeing the OB a lot, so proximity is important. When is the office open? Do they have evening and weekend hours? When is your primary OB in the office?

4 **Size:** Do you prefer a large or small practice? A large practice may offer better hours and more on-site services such as ultrasound and lab testing; it may also be more impersonal and may decrease the chance that your doctor will be on call—and deliver your baby—when you go into labor. Be sure to meet all the OBs in the practice during your pregnancy and be certain you feel comfortable with all of them.

5 **Responsiveness:** How easy is it to get through to the office on the phone? In an emergency, will you be able to reach an OB in your practice at any time of the day or night? How are routine questions handled? How does the office respond when the doctor is running behind schedule? Does the staff notify the patients by phone?

6 **Support staff:** Is the staff knowledgeable and friendly?

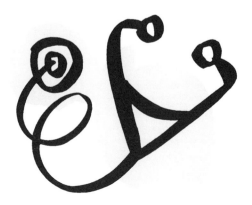

If you have special needs (you have a serious medical condition or are expecting more than one baby), make sure your OB is qualified and experienced to handle your situation or consider signing on with a Maternal and Fetal Medicine specialist. Also, make sure your chosen hospital is equipped to handle your special needs: For example, you may require a level III neonatal intensive care unit or an on-site blood bank.

DEMEANOR

If this is your first pregnancy, you're likely to have more questions and be more uncertain about many issues, from weight gain to amniocentesis. Look for an OB who patiently answers your questions, treats your concerns with sensitivity, gives simple but complete explanations, and doesn't rush visits. Also, consider whether you prefer a doctor who will express strong opinions or whether you'd like someone to help you make your own decisions.

PHILOSOPHY

Even if this is your first pregnancy, you may have strong feelings about issues such as prenatal testing and natural childbirth. Does your OB share, or at least support (whenever possible), your opinions and your Birthing Plan?

Once you've chosen a practice, follow these tips to foster a strong relationship with your OB:

1   **Educate yourself.** Read books on pregnancy and delivery. Ask your OB lots of questions but don't view your doctor as your only resource. Form opinions on matters of importance to you, solicit your OB's judgment, then make your own decisions whenever possible.

2   **Rely on your OB's medical expertise.** There may come a time, due to a complication, when your picture-perfect idea of "how it's going to be" will need to change. Trust your OB to make the right decisions for you and your baby's health.

3 **Respect your OB's time.** Bring your (and the baby's father's) family health history to the first visit (fill out the Health History form in this chapter). Make sure you understand and write down instructions so you're not calling later for reminders. Call your OB with urgent issues but save questions that can wait (jot them down on your next OB Visit form or speak to your OB's nurse).

Do voice concerns and complaints as they arise, so you can resolve issues promptly. If, despite your best efforts, the relationship is simply not working out to your satisfaction, it may be time to leave your OB's practice. Talk to your insurance carrier ahead of time to determine how they will handle this change; sign up with a new OB, then call to have your records transferred. Ideally, place a courtesy call to your OB to explain why you're leaving. He or she should appreciate your candor and value the opportunity to improve the practice.

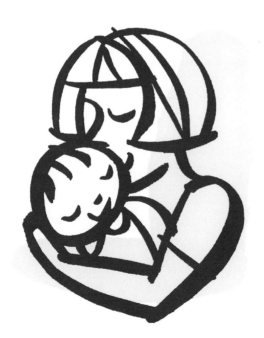

MOM-TO-BE'S HEALTH HISTORY

DATE OF BIRTH

CHILDHOOD ILLNESSES

HOSPITALIZATIONS/OPERATIONS

FERTILITY/PREGNANCY HISTORY

BIRTH CONTROL HISTORY

FIRST DAY OF LAST PERIOD   DATE OF POSITIVE PREGNANCY TEST

GYNECOLOGICAL COMPLICATIONS *(e.g. cysts, fibroids)*

BLOOD TYPE/RH FACTOR FOR BABY'S MOTHER   FOR BABY'S FATHER

ALLERGIES

BLOOD TRANSFUSIONS

OTHER

Note any incidence of the following among baby's parents, siblings, aunts/ uncles, and grandparents.

ALCOHOL, DRUG, AND TOBACCO USE

ANEMIA

ASTHMA

AUTOIMMUNE ILLNESSES OR DEFICIENCIES (E.G. LUPUS)

BIRTH DEFECTS (E.G. CLEFT LIP, CLUBBED FOOT, HEART DEFECTS)

CANCER

CLOTTING DISORDER

DIABETES

GENETIC DISEASE (E.G. CYSTIC FIBROSIS, TAY-SACHS, SICKLE CELL)

HIGH BLOOD PRESSURE

HEART PROBLEMS

KIDNEY DISEASE

MENTAL RETARDATION

SEIZURES

SEXUALLY TRANSMITTED DISEASES

THALASSEMIA

THYROID DISEASE

OTHER

POTENTIAL OBSTETRICIANS

NAME   PHONE

RECOMMENDED BY

NOTES

NAME   PHONE

RECOMMENDED BY

NOTES

NAME   PHONE

RECOMMENDED BY

NOTES

● ◦ ◦ OBSTETRICIAN INTERVIEW

If you were unclear about the office staff responses to some of the basic requirement questions outlined at the beginning of the chapter, feel free to discuss these further with the OB. Otherwise, stick to more sub-stantive questions such as the ones outlined below.

BACKGROUND

- What is your education and training? Are you state-licensed and board-certified?
- How many years have you been in practice? What about the other OBs in your group?
- What are your personal scientific interests? How do you keep up with current medical literature?

PHILOSOPHY

What is your philosophy of care regarding these issues:

- Frequency of appointments
- Routine and level II ultrasounds (number, timing, location)
- Other prenatal testing (options, timing, location)
- Suggested weight gain
- Restrictions regarding food, drink, exercise, work, hair coloring/permanents, travel, sexual intercourse
- Conditions requiring bed rest or other special care

LABOR AND DELIVERY

- When do you arrive at the hospital? Who delivers my baby if you're away? Will I meet all the doctors in the practice and can I request that a doctor I'm not comfortable with not deliver my baby?
- Under what conditions would you induce my baby? Perform a c-section? What is your c-section rate?
- How do you feel about pain management during labor?
- Do you routinely perform episiotomies?

- Whom do you allow in the delivery room? Is that different for a c-section?
- Can we videotape/photograph the birth? Listen to music of our choosing?
- How do you monitor my recovery after the birth?

THE NEXT STEP

How do I sign on with you? When do you recommend I come in for a first appointment?

NOTES

OBSTETRICIAN BASICS

PRIMARY OB'S NAME

OTHER DOCTORS IN THE PRACTICE

OTHER STAFF IN THE PRACTICE

MAIN PHONE NUMBER

OTHER NUMBERS

ADDRESS/DIRECTIONS/PARKING

OFFICE HOURS

EMERGENCY PROCEDURE/OTHER INSTRUCTIONS

● ● ● HEALTH INSURANCE BASICS

HEALTH INSURANCE PLAN

TYPE OF PLAN

PRIMARY MEMBER

MEMBER SOCIAL SECURITY NUMBER

GROUP NUMBER

ID NUMBER

PHONE NUMBER

OTHER NUMBERS

ADDRESS TO SEND CLAIMS TO

OTHER

● ● ● OBSTETRICIAN VISITS

DATE	TIME

DOCTOR

QUESTIONS TO ASK

TEST RESULTS/NOTES

DATE	TIME

DOCTOR

QUESTIONS TO ASK

TEST RESULTS/NOTES

DATE	TIME

DOCTOR

QUESTIONS TO ASK

TEST RESULTS/NOTES

DATE	TIME

DOCTOR

QUESTIONS TO ASK

TEST RESULTS/NOTES

DATE	TIME

DOCTOR

QUESTIONS TO ASK

TEST RESULTS/NOTES

DATE	TIME

DOCTOR

QUESTIONS TO ASK

TEST RESULTS/NOTES

DATE	TIME

DOCTOR

QUESTIONS TO ASK

TEST RESULTS/NOTES

DATE	TIME

DOCTOR

QUESTIONS TO ASK

TEST RESULTS/NOTES

DATE	TIME

DOCTOR

QUESTIONS TO ASK

TEST RESULTS/NOTES

● ● ● OBSTETRICIAN CALLS

DATE	

DOCTOR/NURSE ....

QUESTIONS ....
....

NOTES ....
....
....

DATE	

DOCTOR/NURSE ....

QUESTIONS ....
....

NOTES ....
....
....

DATE	

DOCTOR/NURSE ....

QUESTIONS ....
....

NOTES ....
....
....

DATE

DOCTOR/NURSE

QUESTIONS

NOTES

DATE

DOCTOR/NURSE

QUESTIONS

NOTES

DATE

DOCTOR/NURSE

QUESTIONS

NOTES

● ○ ● PRENATAL TESTING

Record results of tests such as alpha-fetal-protein, ultrasound, amnio-centesis, and CVS.

DATE	# WEEKS

TEST

PROVIDER

RESULTS/NOTES

DATE	# WEEKS

TEST

PROVIDER

RESULTS/NOTES

DATE	# WEEKS

TEST

PROVIDER

RESULTS/NOTES

● ○ ● INSURANCE RECORDS

Stay on top of medical expenses by tracking payments made by you or your insurance carrier for all obstetrical services.

DATE OF SERVICE	PROVIDER	DESCRIPTION OF SERVICE	FEE	CO-PAY	INSURANCE PAYMENT	BALANCE DUE	PAYMENT MADE

● ○ ● INSURANCE CALL LOG

Record dates, names, agreements, and next steps from billing-related
conversations with your insurance carrier and obstetrical providers.

SHOPPING
FOR MOM

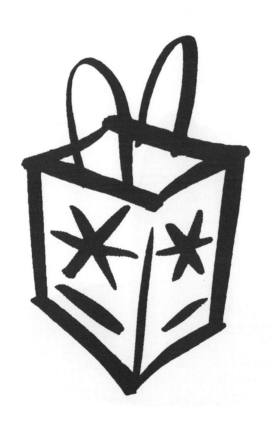

● ◦ ● REAL MOM TIPS: SHOPPING FOR MATERNITY CLOTHING

A maternity store can feel like a very exclusive club; you've earned your membership, so enjoy it. While you thrill at your expanding belly, however, you may not love all the changes your body is going through. Some women glow and feel more "womanly" while they're pregnant, while others can't wait to ditch the big tops and wear a slim belt again. Do what makes you feel your best, whether it's buying a few "I feel like a million bucks" maternity outfits or treating yourself to weekly manicures.

For those of you ready to take the plunge, here are proven tips from veteran maternity shoppers...

GO BEYOND MATERNITY STORES

You have more options than ever when it comes to finding affordable, stylish, comfortable pregnancy wear. The ideal is still maternity clothing, which is designed to suit your changing shape and may make you look and feel your best. But don't assume you need to pay maternity store prices: Shop in maternity outlets, consignment stores, and second-hand children's shops for pregnancy wear at a fraction of the cost. Some women just buy regular clothing in larger sizes while oversize clothes make other women feel like they're wearing a big tent. Decide for yourself. Check out product information books and catalogs in the RESOURCES chapter; consult your phone book for local maternity stores as well as department stores that carry maternity wear.

BORROW, BORROW, BORROW

Ask to borrow maternity clothes from friends and family members. These specialty garments are usually sitting unused in a closet and most moms are happy to lend them out. Keep track on the Borrowed Items log later in this chapter and make sure to return the items in the same condition you found them, freshly laundered or dry-cleaned, with a thank-you note and a small token of appreciation such as a scented hand cream or pretty soaps.

Some women, particularly those requiring professional wear, form maternity clothing exchanges. They pool their maternity wardrobes and lend the collection out to whomever is expecting in the group. This works best, of course, if everyone in the group is in the same size range and pregnant at different times.

Your husband can also be a great resource, particularly in the early months. Raid his closet for button-down shirts, sweats, sweaters, vests, T-shirts, and pj's. Buy decorative clips at a maternity store to cinch back big tops in the early months.

GO FOR CLASSICS

Assuming you'll want to get more use out of your maternity clothes in future pregnancies, go easy on trendy items. Buy classic, timeless pieces that won't go out of style. Choose one solid neutral color for basics like pants and skirts (black, chocolate, or navy, whatever looks best on you); accessorize with colorful tops, scarves, and jewelry. Look for the Pregnancy Survival Kit in department stores or on Web sites; this "wardrobe in a box" includes stretchy maternity pants, skirt, tunic, and a dress that you can mix and match to create different outfits.

GET COMFORTABLE

You'll find it harder to stay comfortable as your body changes in new and different ways. Don't add to that discomfort with binding or ill-fitting clothing. In the early months, as your waist is thickening, use the rubber band trick to get some wear out of your favorite pants or skirts: Simply thread an elastic band into the buttonhole and loop both ends around the button. You may also find your bust line expanding fast; don't skimp on comfortable maternity bras.

Later in the pregnancy, buy items with plenty of stretch to grow and move with your new body. While maternity jeans or khakis may help you feel "normal," you won't get much wear out of them if you dread the thought of putting them on. Maternity stores usually have pregnancy pillows you can try on along with the clothing to help you predict fit and comfort in later months. Test clothes out before making a purchase by sitting, stretching, and bending in the fitting room. Your feet may also grow during pregnancy as a result of stretching ligaments and fluid retention.

Make sure you have at least one pair of comfortable flat shoes with a stacked heel and good arch support. Keep in mind that you may have a tendency to heat up quickly with your hormones in overdrive: Layer clothing so you can peel it off as needed and don't invest in too many sweaters or outerwear.

TIME IT RIGHT

Don't go on a maternity shopping spree too early, when your body is just beginning to expand; you may grow out of a size and need to upgrade when you "pop" at 4 or 5 months. If you want to get the maximum wear out of maternity clothing, however, don't wait until the very end to go shopping, either. Ideally, wear your own looser clothing in the first couple of months, buy a few maternity or larger items at 3 or 4 months, then come back at 5 or 6 months for the home stretch. In any case, look for maternity clothing with ties, clips, and cinches for maximum versatility and wear as your belly expands.

When purchasing through a catalog, maternity store, or Web site, get a good understanding of their sizing. In general, maternity sizes correspond to your pre-pregnancy size. So if you wore a 10 or a medium, those should be your sizes in maternity clothing (if you're carrying multiples, you may need to go up a size or two). Everyone gains weight and carries a pregnancy differently, however, which is one more reason to shop in waves as you see how your body changes.

MATERNITY CLOTHING

Everyday Basics

✓	ITEM	REAL MOM TIPS
○	**6–12 pairs of maternity underwear**	Go for comfort: A cotton/lycra blend will stretch with your expanding belly. Buy a week's worth in your second trimester but be prepared to upgrade to a larger size in your third trimester. The smaller size will also come in handy for the first couple of weeks after the birth, when your waist will still be swollen and you might experience some bleeding. Try under-the-belly and over-the-belly styles to see which you prefer. Some women find regular underwear in larger sizes is cheaper and just as comfortable.
○	**2 maternity bras**	Look for a non-binding stretchy cotton fabric, wide adjustable straps, several back hooks to accommodate your growing bust line, and adequate support. You can also look for these same qualities in a non-maternity or sports bra. Buy new bras as soon as you grow out of your current ones, and upgrade the size as needed. If you plan on breast-feeding, switch to nursing bras in your third trimester instead of buying more maternity bras (see the Nursing checklist later in this chapter).
○	**1–2 sleep bras**	Some women with a larger bust welcome the light support these soft bras provide at night.
○	**2 sleepwear items**	An oversize T-shirt or nightshirt will do the trick (raid your partner's closet).
○	**Bathrobe**	A large, soft bathrobe is ideal.

✓ ITEM	REAL MOM TIPS
○ **2–4 pairs of leggings**	You could live in these! Choose a comfortable stretchy cotton fabric in a solid neutral color. Try both styles—the type that cradles your belly or the kind that stretches over it—to determine which is best for you.
○ **Pair of jeans or khakis**	If you want a more tailored look, these give you style and comfort thanks to a stretchy cotton belly panel.
○ **Pair of overalls**	Many moms-to-be swear by these waist-less, binding-free wonders.
○ **4–8 tops**	Maternity tops and button-down shirts in stretchy fabrics that can be gathered or tied in back are most versatile.
○ **2–4 pairs of maternity support hose**	Particularly useful for women who stand all day, support hose can ease swelling and leg pain.
○ **Maternity support belt**	This helps support your lower back and lift your belly, providing relief for some expectant mothers, especially petite women or those expecting multiples. Check with your OB.
○ **Exercise wear**	Pair loose shorts or maternity bike shorts with a long T-shirt and sweatshirt. Invest in a good sports bra with plenty of support.
○ **Support shoes**	Comfortable, athletic shoes with good arch support are a must.

For Cold-Weather Pregnancies

✔ ITEM	REAL MOM TIPS
○ **2 sweaters or sweatshirts**	Maternity sweaters can be expensive, so consider oversize men's or women's sweaters and sweatshirts.
○ **Jacket or coat**	Don't invest in an expensive coat you'll only wear for a few months. Again, borrow maternity outerwear from a friend or buy a fashionable wool wrap/cape you'll continue to use after the delivery.

For Warm-Weather Pregnancies

✔ ITEM	REAL MOM TIPS
○ **2–4 light tops**	Consider A-line T-shirts and sleeveless button-down shirts for lighter coverage.
○ **2–3 pairs of shorts**	Stretchy cotton is best.
○ **1–2 jumpers**	All the advantages of an overall in a shorter, lightweight version.
○ **1–2 sundresses**	The ultimate in comfort on a hot day, with no binding anywhere. If you buy non-maternity dresses, make sure hemlines are long enough to cover your belly as it grows.
○ **Swimsuit**	Choose a one-piece stretchy tank with adequate breast and belly support. Skirted swimwear does a great job of covering up thighs, too.

Office and Formal Wear

✓ ITEM	REAL MOM TIPS
○ **2–3 basic pants or skirts**	Choose these in neutral colors you can pair with various tops for a different look every day.
○ **4–6 tops**	Use a combination of maternity blouses, button-down shirts, and knit tops.
○ **Blazer**	Select a blazer in a neutral color that coordinates with your pants and skirts.
○ **Formal dress (only if needed)**	This is a good item to borrow. Consider coordinating a nice black skirt with a dressier top. You may also need maternity hosiery.

✓ ITEM	REAL MOM TIPS
○ **Lotion**	There's no proof that lotions or vitamin E reduce the likelihood of stretch marks, but they can soothe the itchy dry skin of your belly.

✓ ITEM	REAL MOM TIPS
○ **Water bottle**	Stay hydrated at all times. Talk to your OB about minimum daily water consumption and make sure you meet those requirements.
○ **Saltines**	Carry these (or whatever foods work for you) if you're experiencing nausea.
○ **Healthy snacks**	Dried fruit or granola bars will tide you over when you get sudden hunger pangs.

✓	ITEM	REAL MOM TIPS
○	**Maternity pillow**	You could purchase or borrow this long pillow to provide full body support while sleeping, or just work with several pillows. In either case, you may wish to buy extra pillows if you don't want to move them every time you roll over in bed.
○	**Prenatal vitamins**	Consult your OB.

NOTES

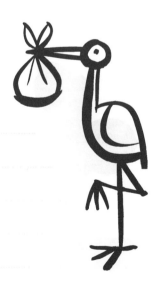

SOOTHERS

✓ ITEM	REAL MOM TIPS
○ **Squirt bottle**	The hospital will probably give you one of these to irrigate your stitches every time you urinate. You can also purchase one at a drugstore.
○ **Sanitary pads**	Necessary for postpartum bleeding.
○ **Hand-held shower**	Another way to irrigate your stitches while in the shower.
○ **Plastic sitz bath**	Yet another vaginal soother. The hospital may give you one to take home. Sitting in a luke-warm bath provides the same effect.
○ **Inflatable doughnut**	This makes sitting much more comfortable the first week after you give birth. Ask if your hospital will let you keep one.
○ **Hemorrhoid cream**	Ask your OB for an over-the counter recom-mendation or a prescription, if necessary.

NURSING

You'll find specifics on breast pumps in the SHOPPING FOR BABY *chapter.*

✓ ITEM	REAL MOM TIPS
○ **2–4 nursing bras**	Make sure they're comfortable and support-ive, and provide easy access via snap panels. Buy these during your last trimester as your breasts reach close to their full size, and go up one size more to accomodate your milk coming in.

✓	ITEM	REAL MOM TIPS
○	**4–8 nursing tops**	These are tailored to allow easy yet discreet access to your breasts for nursing and may be worth the investment should you plan on nursing for several months or more.
○	**6–12 nursing pads**	The washable cotton ones are best. Keep a sweater or jacket on hand in case of an unexpected leak-through.
○	**2–3 nursing nightgowns**	These are not as essential since you'll have more privacy in your home to lift up a T-shirt or unbutton your pj's.
○	**Privacy nursing blanket**	It's hard to maneuver breastfeeding in public, especially in the beginning. This will provide the needed coverage.
○	**Nursing stool**	This stool eases muscle strain in your lower back while you're sitting in a chair or glider.
○	**Nursing pillow**	This U-shaped pillow can help you position your baby for breastfeeding (and can be used later to help baby sit up). The right pillow can ease strain on your neck, arms, and shoulders. Or use several regular pillows and find the most comfortable position.
○	**Nursing cream**	For some new moms, just massaging their own breast milk onto nipples and letting them air dry can ease soreness. Others swear by vitamin E capsules, which they break open and spread onto their nipples. If your nipples are extremely sore or cracked, a lanolin-based cream made expressly for new moms can help you continue breastfeeding. Consult with your OB.

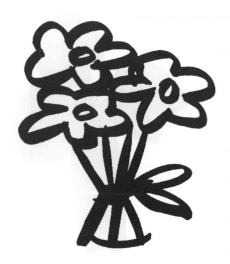

● ● ● BORROWED ITEMS

List items as you borrow them so you'll remember to return them to their proper owner.

ITEM DESCRIPTION   DUE BACK ON

BORROWED FROM   RETURNED ON

ITEM DESCRIPTION   DUE BACK ON

BORROWED FROM   RETURNED ON

ITEM DESCRIPTION   DUE BACK ON

BORROWED FROM   RETURNED ON

ITEM DESCRIPTION   DUE BACK ON

BORROWED FROM   RETURNED ON

ITEM DESCRIPTION   DUE BACK ON

BORROWED FROM   RETURNED ON

ITEM DESCRIPTION   DUE BACK ON

BORROWED FROM   RETURNED ON

ITEM DESCRIPTION

BORROWED FROM

DUE BACK ON

RETURNED ON

ITEM DESCRIPTION

BORROWED FROM

DUE BACK ON

RETURNED ON

ITEM DESCRIPTION

BORROWED FROM

DUE BACK ON

RETURNED ON

ITEM DESCRIPTION

BORROWED FROM

DUE BACK ON

RETURNED ON

ITEM DESCRIPTION

BORROWED FROM

DUE BACK ON

RETURNED ON

ITEM DESCRIPTION

BORROWED FROM

DUE BACK ON

RETURNED ON

SHOPPING
FOR BABY

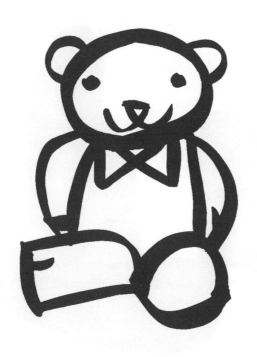

● ● ● REAL MOM TIPS: GEARING UP

So you've seen your doctor, your waist is thickening, you've bought maternity leggings...is this pregnancy starting to feel real yet? Well, get ready, because there's nothing like buying all that Baby Stuff to make it hit home.

Before you buy anything, read this road-tested advice from new moms.

EASE INTO IT

Read over the shopping list, talk to your mom-friends over lunch, visit a baby store or two, and let the information sink in over time. Unless you're a few weeks from your due date, you can afford to take it slowly. Try to enjoy the process. Visualize your nursery as a cozy haven for your newborn baby. Relish taking part in mom-type conversations for the first time. You'll be amazed at how much you'll learn and how soon you'll talk baby equipment like a pro.

FOCUS ON THE ESSENTIALS

Start with the big stuff like nursery furniture, car seat, and stroller; and focus on what you'll need the first few months. This will make preparations a lot more manageable. Clothing and toys are popular baby gifts so you might not want to buy too many of these items until you see what you receive.

ENSURE SAFETY

Look for Juvenile Product Manufacturers Association (JPMA) certification on major items. Send in registration cards so companies can notify you of any recalls or necessary repairs. Check out the THINGS TO DO and RESOURCES chapters for safety and recall information.

BORROW, BORROW, BORROW

Friends who've been there should be happy to lend you baby stuff, but they may not think to offer. So don't be shy...ask! Focus on items that will be of short-lived use like bassinets, bouncer seats, and swings, but accept hand-me-down furniture, strollers, clothing, and toys as well. Just make sure all items measure up to current safety standards (again, refer to the safety and recall info in the RESOURCES chapter for help). While you're at it, start clipping coupons for diapers and other bulk items and stake out your favorite discount superstore. And don't neglect those second-hand baby stores and garage sales: They can be real treasure troves. (But use care when buying cribs or car seats second hand. Safety requirements have changed dramatically in recent years.)

MAKE ROOM

You'll be amazed at how much space baby stuff can take up. Go ahead with that long overdue garage sale—time to let go of that old record collection and those bell bottoms you haven't worn since high school—or you'll soon be tripping over strollers and swings!

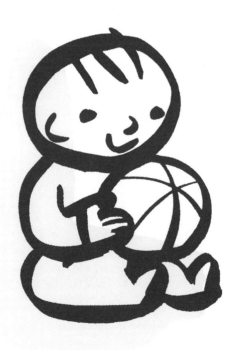

● ● ● CHECKLIST FOR YOUR NEWBORN

This list is designed to be comprehensive, so you don't have to worry about what's missing. (Spaces are provided for your add-ins, just in case.) Must-have's are in caps; the rest is up to you. The range of quantities depends on how often you'll do laundry: the first number assumes you'll do the wash twice a week, the second number once a week. Also, check out all the practical tips from new moms. Turn to the RESOURCES *chapter for catalog and Web site suggestions, safety information, and books that provide in-depth and updated brand comparisons.*

Furniture

✓ I T E M	R E A L M O M T I P S
○ **CRIB**	Look for a side railing that lowers easily and quietly, as well as an adjustable mattress height. Some models convert to toddler beds.
○ **CRIB MATTRESS**	Today's crib mattresses are sold separately from the crib and are almost always waterproof. You can buy foam or coil; either way, make sure it's firm and fits snugly against all sides of the crib.
○ **DRESSER**	You can get a combination dresser and changing table (or put a changing pad on top of a regular dresser) but you'll use the top drawer for diapering supplies, leaving only two drawers for clothes; this is fine if you have extra shelf space in a closet. If you'll be purchasing a separate changing table, any size dresser will do. Smaller drawers are great for socks, hats, and other tiny items.
○ **Changing table**	Look for one with a drawer where you can stash toiletry supplies away from your baby's reach once he or she begins to crawl.

Furniture continued

✔ ITEM	REAL MOM TIPS
○ **Bassinet**	With a bassinet, your baby can sleep in your bedroom for the first few months, which makes 3 a.m. feedings much easier. Try to borrow one, or use a portable crib. Some bassinets have a removable Moses basket, which you can use outside or away from home. Others have a side that opens up to an adult bed, for easy access in the middle of the night.
○ **Rocker or glider**	You need to have somewhere to sit in the nursery and this is a nice, comfortable option. Choose the cushion fabric carefully as you may want to use this rocker/glider for a later baby or move it to a family room.
○ **Nursing stool**	Reduces stress on the lower back when sitting in the rocker or glider. If you don't want to get the expensive ottoman to match the glider, a simple wood stool works fine.
○ **Shelf set**	You'll be amazed at how many children's books you'll collect.
○ **Toy bin or basket**	Make sure wooden bins don't have a lid that can snap shut on little fingers. Soft mesh bins or woven baskets are great.
○ **Adult bed**	Camp out in the nursery on difficult nights and let your partner get a good night's sleep.
○	
○	
○	

For the Crib

✓ ITEM	REAL MOM TIPS
○ **SET OF CRIB BUMPERS**	Bumpers create a cozy environment and prevent little fingers and feet from getting stuck in crib railings.
○ **2–6 FITTED SHEETS**	Buy two for your bassinet (if you have one), and two for the crib. Cotton flannel is nice in cold weather.
○ **2 CRIB BLANKETS**	Buy the appropriate weight for the season: Cotton is soft and washable; fleece is a warm alternative for cold weather (and it's nice to tuck around baby in the stroller, too).
○ **Crib dust ruffles**	A nice touch because a crib can look bare without it. Also, dust ruffles hide items you've stored beneath the crib.
○ **2 mattress pads**	Adds extra cushioning but makes it harder to get a sheet onto the mattress.
○ **1–2 waterproof liners**	Buy one for your bassinet (if you have one), and one for the crib.
○ **Quilts and pillows**	Decorative items for the room, but don't place them in a baby's crib.
○	

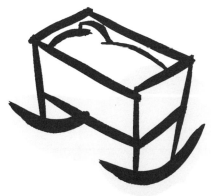

Accessories

✓	ITEM	REAL MOM TIPS
○	**WINDOW TREATMENTS**	Make sure you have room-darkening shades, blinds, or curtains to help baby distinguish between day and night and to facilitate day-time napping.
○	**LIGHTING**	You may need a ceiling or dresser lamp (floor lamps can be knocked over by a crawling baby). Lights with dimmers allow for less disruptive middle-of-the-night diaper changes and feedings.
○	**Night light**	Automatic ones are nice: They come on at night, shut off in the daytime.
○	**Laundry hamper**	You can use a basket, too. A cloth bag insert makes for easy toting.
○	**Closet and drawer organizers**	Closet organizers can give you more shelf space since you won't be hanging much quite yet. Drawer organizers help you keep all those tiny socks and mittens sorted.
○	**6 baby hangers**	To hang bulky or dressy clothing.
○	**Music player**	Choose a mini-stereo, boom box, or cassette-player/nightlight combination.
○		
○		
○		
○		

Buy 100% cotton (soft and breathable), machine-washable items. Prewash all baby clothes you plan to keep because most shrink. Consider newborn sizing only for preemies or small babies since they'll grow out of this size so quickly. Snaps up the front and legs make diaper changes easier.

For All Babies

✔ ITEM	REAL MOM TIPS
○ **3–6 RECEIVING BLANKETS**	Most newborns love to be swaddled.
○ **4–8 BODYSUITS**	Also called Onesies, these T-shirts snap between the legs. Buy them in size small (3–6 months) and layer them under receiving blankets or sleepers. You could also buy side snap or tie T-shirts but they ride up.
○ **4–8 SLEEPERS OR STRETCHIES**	Your newborn will live in these one-piece pj's day and night. The small size (3–6 months) should be fine for the first few months.
○ **2–4 infant gowns (kimonos)**	These look like long nightgowns and make diaper changes a snap, especially in the middle of the night. They come only in newborn sizes. Look for an elastic bottom, without strings or ties that can be choking hazards.
○ **No-scratch baby mittens**	Good if you're reluctant to cut your baby's tiny fingernails and want to prevent scratches. Still, they can be hard to keep on.
○ **3–6 coveralls or rompers for play**	These are like stretchies but without the feet and a little dressier for daytime and excursions. Go for the medium size (6–9 months) since your baby will probably stay In sleepers day and night for the first few months.
○ **1–2 sweaters**	Buy cotton for summer, fleece for winter—both are nice and soft. A cardigan is easier to maneuver in the first few months.

For All Babies *(continued)*

✓ ITEM	REAL MOM TIPS
○ **3–6 pairs of booties or socks**	Use these with non-footed clothing or with a nightgown on chilly nights. Make sure the elastic is not too tight around the ankles.
○ **1–2 outdoor hats**	A wide-brimmed cotton hat or baseball cap is nice for summer, a fleece hat with ear and neck flaps is comfy in winter.
○	
○	

For Cold-Weather Babies

✓ ITEM	REAL MOM TIPS
○ **SNOWSUIT OR BUNTING**	Snowsuits have legs; buntings do not. Snow-suits are more practical for car seats and strollers because of the straps. Get one with a hood for maximum protection from the cold. Fleece is a nice choice for mild fall and winter days.
○ **1–2 blanket sleepers**	These are made with a thicker fleecy material for cold nights and come in legged or easy bag versions.
○ **1–2 infant caps**	A close-fitting cotton cap is nice to layer under a snowsuit hood or to use indoors if your home is on the cool side.
○	
○	

With Disposables

✓	ITEM	REAL MOM TIPS
○	**70 DISPOSABLE DIAPERS**	Buy three packs of newborn size to start—babies grow fast. Expect to use about 10 diapers a day. Find a nearby discount store to purchase diapers and other essentials in bulk.
○	**Diaper pail**	This seals in dirty diaper odors so you're not emptying the trash constantly. Some diaper pails (like the Diaper Genie) require special refill canisters; this gets costly, so use the pail for soiled diapers only.
○	**Small trash can**	If you're using a diaper pail with special refill canisters, line a separate trash can with a small garbage bag and use it for wet diapers (they don't smell much but you'll want to empty the can every few days).

With Cloth Diapers

✓	ITEM	REAL MOM TIPS
○	**35–70 PREFOLDED CLOTH DIAPERS**	If you'll be washing them yourself, assess how often you want to do laundry. A diaper service will usually provide one week's worth (around 70 diapers) and they'll pick up dirty diapers and deliver new ones weekly.
○	**4–8 DIAPER COVERS**	These secure cloth diapers without pins or clips, using velcro. They're machine washable and usually waterproof. You will need to buy larger sizes as your baby grows.

With Cloth Diapers *(continued)*

✓ ITEM	REAL MOM TIPS
○ **DIAPER BIN**	A diaper service can provide this (at an additional cost), including plastic bags and deodorizer refills.
○ **4 diaper pins or clips**	If you decide against the diaper covers, you'll need to secure the cloth diaper onto your baby with two of these. Top the diaper with waterproof pants to protect against leaks.
○ **3 waterproof pants**	Get these if you're using pins or clips. They're machine washable and come in different sizes (trade up as needed).

Either Way

✓ ITEM	REAL MOM TIPS
○ **BOX OF 80–100 BABY WIPES**	Use soft cloth-like paper towels (like Viva) and plain tap water the first few weeks. Once you switch to wipes, buy the unscented, alcohol-free kind. Save money by buying them in a box the first time and then buying refill bags after that. There's no need to use wipes for wet diapers, only soiled ones. Also use wipes to sanitize toys or to clean your hands after a diaper change on the go.
○ **CHANGING PAD**	A waterproof foam pad with elevated sides offers a good spot for diaper changes. You could buy more than one to set up additional changing stations in your home (one station per floor is ideal).

Either Way *(continued)*

✔ ITEM	REAL MOM TIPS
○ **2 CHANGING PAD COVERS**	A terry cover is soft—you don't want baby lying on cold plastic.
○ **4–8 WATERPROOF LAP PADS**	Place one under baby's bottom on the changing pad to minimize cover changes.
○ **Wipes and diaper holder**	Hooks onto the side of most changing tables for easy access.
○ **Wipes warmer**	Wipes can be cool against a little bottom, but your baby will get used to it. If you live in a cold climate, a warm wipe can make diaper changes cozier for your baby.
○	
○	

TOILETRIES

Grooming

✔ ITEM	REAL MOM TIPS
○ **NAIL GROOMING SET**	A set usually comes with nail clippers, baby scissors, and an emery board. See what you feel most comfortable using. Choose a time when baby is relaxed or sleeping to try a manicure for the first time.
○ **Soft brush and comb**	Only if baby has lots of hair.
○ **Baby lotion**	Use lotion on baby's dry skin, especially after a bath and for baby massages.
○	

Bathing

✓ ITEM	REAL MOM TIPS
○ **BOWL FOR WARM WATER**	You'll use this plastic bowl for paper-towel-and-water diaper changes in the first few weeks and for wipe-downs on the changing table.
○ **6–12 BABY WASHCLOTHS**	Use for wipe-downs and baths, as well as to cover your baby boy's penis during diaper changes (watch out for squirting).
○ **BABY BATH TUB**	Both you and baby will feel much more secure using a baby tub instead of the big tub or a kitchen sink. Place the baby tub in a sink rather than an adult bathtub to reduce stress on your back. This is a good item to borrow because you'll stop using it when your baby sits up (at around 6 months).
○ **2–4 HOODED TOWELS**	You could also use regular towels, although the hood is nice to keep baby's head warm.
○ **BABY SHAMPOO**	Make sure it's tear-free.
○ **Baby bath soap**	Water is all you really need to wash a newborn. You could also get a 2-in-1 soap/shampoo (Johnson & Johnson and Baby Magic make them).
○ **Bath toys**	Rubber ducks, vinyl books, balls, etc. It's fun to blow bubbles, too!
○ **Bath toy mesh bag**	Get a bag with suction cups for your bathroom wall. Helps toys air out and dry, and keeps them out of the way.
○	
○	

Laundry

✓	ITEM	REAL MOM TIPS
○	**Baby laundry soap**	Use a mild detergent, such as Dreft or Ivory Snow, to wash all baby clothes, sheets, and towels. You can also use a laundry soap that's free of dyes and perfumes. Avoid dryer sheets unless they're also free of dyes and fragrances.
○	**Pre-wash stain remover**	Like Shout or Spray 'n' Wash. Helps combat tough stains from formula or spit-up, and later on from solid foods.
○		
○		

FEEDING

See the SHOPPING FOR MOM *chapter for the nursing mother's needs.*

If Nursing

✓	ITEM	REAL MOM TIPS
○	**BREAST PUMP**	Let dad and others bottle-feed expressed milk once in a while. Rent an electric model (portable is better) and remember to get the breast pump kit from the hospital.
○	**50 MILK STORAGE BAGS AND STICKERS**	Freezing breast milk is a good way to stock up. Use the stickers to date each bag of pumped milk. Write the date on the sticker and not on the bag directly to avoid ink leaking into the milk.
○	**2 BOTTLES WITH NIPPLES, COLLARS, AND CAPS**	To let others feed baby with expressed milk. See more info in the next checklist on bottle-feeding.

If Bottle-Feeding

✓ ITEM	REAL MOM TIPS
○ **6–10 BOTTLES**	You can buy all 8-oz. or some 4-oz. bottles. You'll eventually just use the 8-oz. size. Newborns feed every 3 to 4 hours and it's nice to have a few bottles ready to go. Baby bottles come in different shapes, all claiming to reduce air ingestion. Try a variety, but you may find the straight bottles work just fine, especially if your baby burps well.
○ **6–10 NIPPLES, COLLARS, AND CAPS**	They come with the bottles. Each bottle brand has a different shape nipple (some are interchangeable), so wait to see which baby prefers before committing. Silicone nipples last longer and don't crack like rubber ones. Start with the slow-flow (stage 1) nipples.
○ **1 WEEK'S SUPPLY OF FORMULA**	As directed by your pediatrician. Powder is cheaper than ready-to-use or liquid concentrate.
○ **Disposable bottle liners**	Some moms swear by this system (by Playtex), which is sanitary and cuts down on bottle cleaning. Others find it's a pain— and you have to wash the nipples anyway.
○ **Bottle of baby water**	Unlike spring water, this water is purified and has fluoride. Use it in emergencies when no boiled water for powdered formula is on hand. Refill the empty bottle (a funnel will help) with cooled boiled water for future use.
○ **Plastic pitcher with lid**	To make powdered formula in quantity. Look for a 2- to 3-quart pitcher with a pour spout. You'll need a measuring cup and a whisk as well.
○ **Dishwasher basket**	A must for nipples if you're using a dishwasher. The big basket without compartments is easiest.

If Bottle-Feeding (continued)

☑ I T E M	R E A L M O M T I P S
○ **Bottle/nipple drying and storage rack**	Put it on your kitchen counter with a paper towel underneath to let bottles and nipples air out.
○ **Bottle sterilizer**	You'll use this if you don't have a dishwasher. You can also boil bottles and nipples in a large pot of water and remove them with tongs.
○ **Bottle/nipple brush**	To clean out dried-up formula. Not necessary if you're using a dishwasher.
○ **Bottle warmer**	Some models keep a bottle cold then heat it when needed—handy for middle-of-the night feedings if your kitchen is not near your nursery. Make sure your chosen bottles fit into your brand of bottle warmer.

FEEDING

Either Way

☑ I T E M	R E A L M O M T I P S
○ **6–12 BURP CLOTHS**	No need to buy fancy ones; cloth diapers work just fine.
○ **3–6 bibs**	Cloth bibs are best for spit-up or drool. Bibs that slip over the head or secure with velcro are easier to use than bibs that tie. You could also tuck a cloth diaper under baby's chin (the regular, not the prefolded variety, works best).
○	

Toys

✓ ITEM	REAL MOM TIPS
○ **Bouncer seat**	Great place to park baby so you can watch him/her while you're eating dinner or taking a shower. The seat bounces only with baby's movement. Options include battery-operated vibration, toy bar, and sun canopy. Stop using the seat when baby pulls forward because it could tip over.
○ **Swing**	Very soothing to many babies. Buy one that's battery-operated so there's no need to crank it and get one with several speeds if possible. Look for a sturdy frame, secure restraints, and a padded seat. A reclining feature is nice for a young baby.
○ **Mobile for changing station**	This is a nice distraction for a squirmy baby. You'll need to hang it from the wall or ceiling because it will be too low and unstable when clamped onto the side of the changing table.
○ **Mobile for crib**	Go for bright colors, three-dimensional shapes, and a pleasant lullaby. This should attach securely to the side of the crib. Remove it when baby can sit up (at about 6 months).
○ **Crib activity center**	A soft cloth version is ideal to start. Baby can remove plush animals, rattles, and teethers for play. Be sure it's securely attached to crib railings.
○ **Activity gym**	Like the Gymini. This arch features dangling toys for your baby to gaze and touch while lying on his/her back. Buy extra rings to drop toys closer to baby or place baby in C-shaped pillow under the gym.

✓ ITEM	REAL MOM TIPS
○ **Play/activity mat**	Soft mat with different designs, colors, textures, and sounds to stimulate a baby lying on his/her stomach.
○ **C-shaped pillow**	Like the Boppy. This props up a baby, offering a new vantage point. Provides support for an older baby who's learning to sit.
○ **Developmental toys**	Like the Lamaze or Kids II/Discovery line of toys. Great gift idea when family and friends ask what to get your child.
○ **Stuffed animals, puppets, dolls**	Some babies will like them right away, others won't enjoy these for a few more months. Get small ones they can hold onto early on.
○ **Rattles and squeaky toys**	Look for a variety of shapes, colors, textures, and sounds. Soft ones prevent accidental bumps in the first months.
○ **2 pacifiers**	Go for silicone instead of rubber, which dries out and cracks. Try different shapes and sizes to determine baby's preference before investing in several of the same kind.
○ **Pacifier holder**	No more dropped or lost pacifiers! The cord attaches to the pacifier and clips onto baby's clothing. (Do not use unattended.)
○ **Music**	Collections of lullabies and play songs are great on tape or CD.
○ **Books**	Look for board books with bright colors, big pictures, fun sounds, and interesting textures.
○	
○	

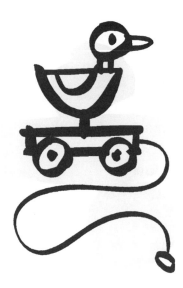

SAFETY

See safety information in the THINGS TO DO *chapter for extensive coverage of this topic.*

✔ ITEM	REAL MOM TIPS
○ **Baby monitor**	Get a model with a lights display as well so you can "hear" baby even over TV or vacuum noise. Use it in an outlet instead of replacing batteries all the time, or look for a rechargeable model. Test the monitor out for clear reception and exchange it for a different type if there's too much static or interference with your phone line. An intercom feature comes in handy in a multi-level home.
○ **Pager**	Get one for your labor coach when you're in your last trimester. Keep it after the birth for whenever you're away from baby (a great way to reach you at the movies, for example).
○	
○	

Basics

✓ ITEM	REAL MOM TIPS
○ **MEDICAL REFERENCE BOOK**	See the RESOURCES chapter for recommendations.
○ **RECTAL THERMOMETER**	This is the temperature reading pediatricians prefer since it's most accurate. Underarm or ear thermometers can be tricky to operate with accuracy. Check with your pediatrician.
○ **PETROLEUM JELLY**	To help circumcisions heal and to apply to the tip of the rectal thermometer before insertion.
○ **STERILE COTTON**	To clean a newborn baby's eyes and wipe a bottom recovering from a diaper rash.
○ **COTTON SWABS**	To apply rubbing alcohol to the umbilical cord stub and ointment to cuts.
○ **STERILE GAUZE PADS**	To help in healing baby's circumcision and to clean dirty scrapes.
○ **TWEEZERS**	To remove splinters.
○ **RUBBING ALCOHOL OR ALCOHOL PADS**	To clean baby's umbilical cord stub, disinfect the rectal thermometer and tweezers.
○ **HYDROGEN PEROXIDE**	To clean abrasions and cuts.
○ **ANTIBIOTIC OINTMENT**	Like Neosporin. To help prevent infection in minor cuts and scrapes.
○ **DIAPER RASH OINTMENT**	To help in healing a diaper rash. Look for brands like Desitin with zinc oxide for maximum protection. Use it at the first sign of redness and keep the area dry with frequent diaper changes.
○ **CALAMINE LOTION**	To cool sunburn, heat, and other rashes, as well as itchy bug bites.

✓	ITEM	REAL MOM TIPS
○	**INFANT ORAL MEDICINE DROPPER OR SYRINGE**	To measure medications.
○	**INFANT NASAL ASPIRATOR**	To help clear out baby's stuffy nose.
○	**SALINE NOSE DROPS**	To lubricate baby's nasal passages.
○	**Sterile adhesive bandages**	To protect small cuts and abrasions. For older, mobile babies.
○	**Non-stick bandage roll**	To wrap around a larger wound. For older, mobile babies.
○	**Roll of first-aid adhesive tape**	To hold non-stick bandages in place. For older, mobile babies.
○	**Small ice pack**	To relieve pain and reduce swelling of minor bumps and bruises.
○	**Cornstarch baby powder**	To help keep skin cool and dry in warm weather. Never use talc, which can be dangerous if inhaled.
○	**Antibacterial liquid soap**	Place a bottle beside each sink for frequent hand washing.
○	**Humidifier**	Dry air in cold weather is tough on baby's little nose; a humidifier can help. Make sure it uses cold water (hot water is a scalding hazard) and follow all maintenance recommendations.
○		
○		
○		

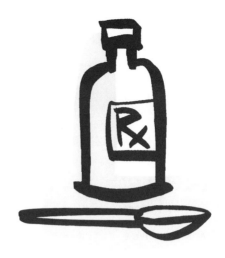

MEDICINE CABINET

Administer Only as Directed by a Pediatrician

✓	ITEM	REAL MOM TIPS
○	**SYRUP OF IPECAC**	Induces vomiting, for use in some cases of poisoning.
○	**ORAL REHYDRATION SOLUTION**	Like Pedialyte. Helps hydrate a baby with diarrhea or who is vomiting.
○	**INFANT ACETAMINOPHEN**	Like Baby Tylenol. Helps reduce pain and fever.
○	**Cough & cold medicine**	Like Pediacare.
○	**Vitamin supplement**	Like Trivisol with iron. May be needed if baby is on a low-iron formula, breastfed, or premature.
○	**Gas relief drops**	Like Mylicon.
○	**Teething gel**	Like Orajel.
○	**Baby oil**	For cradle cap. Your pediatrician may also recommend a medicated shampoo.
○	**Sun block**	Make sure it's at least SPF 15 and blocks both UVA and UVB rays.

Basics

✓	ITEM	REAL MOM TIPS
○	**Diaper bag**	The backpack version keeps your arms and hands free. Forego a cutesy print for something more unisex that even dad won't mind carrying. Choose a sturdy washable fabric with lots of pockets. Make sure a changing pad comes with it.
○	**Travel case for wipes**	Thin case to carry a few baby wipes along.
○	**Bottle cooler bag**	Put a cold pack in this zippered pouch and keep your bottles and gel teething rings cold.
○	**1–2 cold packs**	Keep small cold packs in the freezer and pop them into the cooler bag as needed.
○	**Powdered formula container**	This is a nifty gadget with compartments for pre-measured powder. Bring along a bottle of water, dump in the powder, shake it up, and a nice room-temperature bottle is ready for baby. Some specialty bottles also have separate chambers for water and powder, so you can easily mix them together when it's time for a feeding.
○		
○		
○		
○		
○		

For the Car

✓ ITEM	REAL MOM TIPS
○ **CAR SEAT**	By law your child cannot ride in a car without one. Get a convertible car seat that will face backwards (for babies up to 20 lbs and until 1 year old) and forward (20 to 40 lbs. and 1 to 4 years old). An infant car seat (up to 20 lbs., rear-facing only) is nice for a small baby and doubles as an infant carrier. Get it with a base that's permanently installed in your car for easy removal. If you buy a Snap 'n Go frame, this becomes your stroller, too.
○ **HEAD SUPPORTS**	Support a newborn's unsteady head. Get several for the car seat, swing, and stroller, as needed.
○ **Sun shades**	If you install your car seat by a rear seat window, you may need shades to protect your baby from the sun. The easiest to use secure to the window with suction cups.
○ **Car seat protector**	Goes under the car seat to protect the car's cloth/leather seat from marks and spills.
○ **Car seat toy and activity center**	Helps amuse baby on long car rides, especially when he/she is facing backwards and is too small to look out the window.
○ **Rear-facing seat mirror**	A small mirror that attaches to the back seat, seat headrest, or window lets you see your baby's reflection in your rearview mirror.
○	
○	

For Travel

✅ ITEM	REAL MOM TIPS
○ **Portable crib/ playpen**	Like the Pack 'n Play. Make sure to get one that folds easily and compactly, and unfolds securely. It's handy if a carrying case with a shoulder strap is included. You could borrow this when needed unless you use it often.
○ **2 portable crib sheets**	Pack these so your baby's not sleeping on vinyl.
○ **Car seat travel tote**	Protects your car seat if you check it in at the airport.
○ **Stroller travel tote**	Protects your stroller if you check it in at the airport (not necessary if you check it in at the gate).
○	
○	

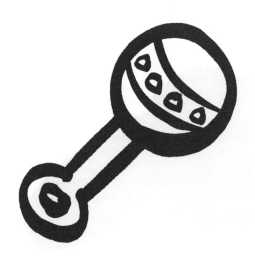

For Walks

✔ ITEM	REAL MOM TIPS
○ **STROLLER**	Assess your needs. A carriage or pram is nice for a sleeping newborn but you won't use it for long (so it's a great item to borrow). An umbrella stroller is lightweight and folds, so it's ideal for travel and to keep in the car trunk. A jogging stroller is sturdy and gives you and your baby the most comfortable ride, but it takes up a lot of space. Look for a stroller that does double duty. The stroller/car seat combination (Snap'n Go) is great for air travel—you wheel the stroller up to the gate, take the car seat on the plane, and check in the stroller frame at the gate where it will be waiting for you on your arrival. (This only works with infant car seats, so you'll need a different stroller when you switch to a regular car seat.) Other strollers convert from a carriage to a sturdy full-size stroller. Overall, look for a seat that's padded and reclines, particularly for a newborn. You'll need a canopy and a roomy storage basket. Test drive the stroller to make sure you're comfortable with the handle height and ease of stride.
○ **Soft baby carrier or sling**	A great way to carry your baby while keeping your arms free. A sling like Nojo cradles a newborn baby up to 3 months. A front baby carrier like Baby Bjorn or Snugli carries baby upright, facing in (up to 3 months) or out (after 3 months).
○ **Stroller pad**	An additional cushiony layer for a hard umbrella stroller seat.
○ **Stroller weather shield**	Vented plastic cover to protect baby on rainy, snowy, or windy days.

For Walks *(continued)*

✓	ITEM	REAL MOM TIPS
○	**Stroller mesh bag**	Get this if your stroller does not come with storage under or behind the seat—you'll need the cargo space.
○	**Stroller toy/play bar**	Entertains baby on long walks.
○	**Sunglasses**	Adorable, if your baby will keep them on.
○		
○		
○		

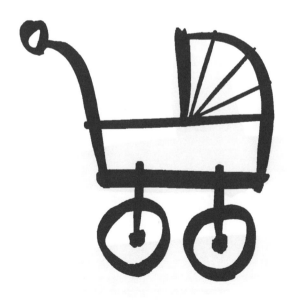

✓ I T E M	R E A L M O M T I P S
○ **Announcements**	Get the envelopes early so you can address and stamp them before your baby's arrival. If you've chosen custom-printed announcements, select the design before the birth, then call in the baby information from the hospital (see the BACK HOME chapter).
○ **Thank-you cards**	Cards that match the announcements are a nice touch.
○ **Stamps**	Buy extra so you have them on hand for thank-you notes.
○ **Camera**	Don't forget extra film and batteries.
○ **Video camera**	Make sure you have extra tape and that your battery is recharged.
○ **Photo storage box**	Stores photo negatives, extra pictures, and thicker items like baby's hospital cap or ID bracelet.
○ **Baby photo album**	Don't wait too long to put your baby's album together. Pick out your favorite pictures as you go and note the date or baby's age on the back. It's amazing how quickly you'll forget.
○ **Baby scrapbook and diary**	Make sure to record all of your baby's firsts, from first smile to first tooth to first step.
○ **Book on infant care**	See the RESOURCES chapter for recommendations.
○	
○	
○	

CHECKLIST FOR YOUR OLDER BABY (4 TO 6 MONTHS)

CLOTHING

✓ ITEM	REAL MOM TIPS
○ 4–8 BODYSUITS	Onesies in larger sizes are essential now, to use as undergarments in cold weather or to double as nightwear in the summer.
○ 4–8 PLAY OUTFITS	One-piece rompers or overalls with snaps at the legs make for easier diaper changes. Buy larger sizes because cotton shrinks and babies grow fast.
○ 4–8 NIGHT CLOTHES	Blanket sleepers with legs are great for crawling babies (who kick off their blankets) in cold weather. Use lighter sleepers or stretchies the rest of the year. Onesies will do the trick in warm weather.
○ OUTERWEAR	Keep on hand soft cotton or fleece sweaters, hats, mittens, jackets, coats, and snowsuits and use as needed.
○ FOOTWEAR	Socks or booties to keep toes warm on cool days.
○ Swimwear	Pair a swimsuit with a disposable swim diaper and a wide-brimmed hat. A baby pool is ideal once your infant can sit up, but never leave your baby unattended in or near water.
○	

✔ ITEM	REAL MOM TIPS
○ **BATH SEAT**	When your baby can sit up, this keeps him or her upright while giving you free hands to lather, shampoo, and play.
○ **Shampoo visor**	When baby can sit up, if he/she will keep it on, this can keep suds out of eyes.

✔ ITEM	REAL MOM TIPS
○ **TOOTHBRUSH**	Use a baby toothbrush when your baby's first tooth comes in.
○ **BABY TOOTHPASTE**	Don't use adult toothpaste because your baby may not be able to digest it (yes, he/she will swallow it). Also, the fluoride in regular toothpaste can permanently stain a baby's teeth.

✔ ITEM	REAL MOM TIPS
○ **HIGH CHAIR**	Look for a sturdy base, adjustable height, a removable seat cover (for easy cleaning), and one-handed tray release. A reclining seat is nice for a young baby.
○ **3–6 BIBS**	Over-the-head or velcro closures are easier than ties. Choose wipe-off plastic or washable thick terry cloth.
○ **2–4 SOFT-COATED SPOONS**	A must to protect baby's delicate gums and new teeth.

ITEM	REAL MOM TIPS
○ **BABY CEREAL**	Start with one grain at a time (rice, oatmeal, barley) to ensure your baby's not allergic.
○ **BABY FOOD IN JARS**	Buy ready-made or make your own. Start with finely pureed one-ingredient veggies and fruits.
○ **Baby food organizer**	Rotating caddies allow for easy access.
○ **Food grinder**	You'll need this if you're making your own baby food to ensure a fine consistency.
○ **Plastic storage containers**	To store leftover baby foods.
○ **2–4 plastic feeding bowls**	Keep the bowl away from curious fingers or they'll tip it over. Buy a bowl that comes with a suction base: Use just the bowl for now, and use the bowl with the base later when your baby starts to self-feed.
○ **2–4 training cups**	The spill-proof feature on these cups requires baby to suck hard so you may not use them until later in the first year.
○ **Waterproof floor mat**	Protects the floor under the high chair from messy spills (just wipe the mat clean). You could also use newspaper and toss it after each meal.
○ **High chair suction toy**	Keep your baby amused while you prepare his or her meal.
○	
○	
○	

✔ ITEM	REAL MOM TIPS
○ **CRIB ACTIVITY CENTER**	Now's the time for a souped-up electronic version with buttons and levers that allow your child to make sounds and light up the toy.
○ **TEETHING TOYS AND RINGS**	Chewing on hard or cold surfaces relieves sore gums. Gel-filled teethers can be stored either in the refrigerator or freezer.
○ **Interactive electronic toys**	Brands like V-Tech have a huge assortment with fun sounds and lights activated by buttons, levers, and wheels. These will keep your baby busy for hours.
○ **Stationary exerciser**	Like the Exersaucer. Controversial due to issues with spinal development if overused, so check with your pediatrician and use sparingly.
○ **Doorway jumper**	Again, controversial. Check with your pediatrician.
○ **More toys**	Stacking cups, blocks, balls, trucks, musical instruments, etc., all entertain while working your baby's fine motor skills.

✔ ITEM	REAL MOM TIPS
○ **Backpack carrier**	Built with a sturdy frame, it supports older babies who are able to sit up. Borrow one to see if you and your child enjoy it before buying.
○ **Travel booster seat**	Folds down compactly, for travel with a baby who can sit up.

● ● ● REAL MOMS-OF-TWINS TIPS

Twins on the way? You are truly doubly blessed. There is something cuter than a baby, and that's two! Ready-made playmates, they will delight (and yes, exhaust) you at every turn; plus, they'll share a unique relationship and a special bond.

Because twins are more likely to be born early, you may be put on bed rest or limited activity, especially in your last trimester. With that in mind, try to get all your essential preparations and purchases done by your sixth month. If you haven't completed your shopping and you're put on bed rest, don't worry; you can shop by phone or Internet so you won't be scrambling for basics when bringing two newborns home. And when it comes to shopping for twins, consider these additional practical tips from mothers of multiples.

NURSERY

Your babies can sleep in the same crib for the first few months until they become too big or too mobile. At 4 or 5 months, they'll each need their own crib. (You can fold back the bumper pads on one side of each crib so they can still see each other.) If you have a narrow nursery, get two cribs with straight headboards or footboards so they can stand end to end. Do get a changing table and a tall chest of drawers. You'll need the extra space.

LAYETTE

How much more clothing will you need? Well, that depends on the sex of your babies. If you're having two of the same flavor, take the smaller quantity from the Checklist for Your Newborn above, and buy 1 ½ times that much (this assumes you're doing laundry at least twice a week). If you're having a boy and a girl, you'll need twice the quantity, unless you buy a lot of unisex clothing. If you don't know what you're having, go the unisex route for now.

You'll need to decide if you wish to dress your cuties alike, especially if you're having two boys or two girls. It really is adorable, although identical twins could benefit from some differentiation. Regardless, take advantage of it now, because you won't be making those decisions for long.

With twins, convenience is critical. Buy items that are easy to wash, wear, and remove. And since your babies are likely to be smaller than average, you may need extra newborn clothing.

DIAPERING

A changing station (a pad and supplies) on each floor is ideal—you don't want to be carrying babies up and down the stairs for every diaper change.

TOILETRIES

Don't buy or borrow two baby bathtubs since you'll be washing only one baby at a time.

FEEDING

If you'll be nursing, get a pump so you can enjoy a break once in a while. Consider a nursing pillow made especially for moms of twins to breastfeed both babies at once (quite tricky, especially in the beginning).

If you choose to bottle-feed, buy powdered formula in bulk and make the day's bottles ahead of time (using the pitcher method). You'll need 1½ to 2 times as many bottles as recommended and will be running the dishwasher daily (invest in one now—it'll be worth it). Two dishwasher baskets (one to collect dirty nipples in the dishwasher, the other to air dry nipples on the counter) and two drying racks (due to the sheer number of bottles you'll have) make sense. A few color bottles are helpful when one baby is sick and you need to keep bottles separate. When bottle-feeding two babies at once, two C-shaped pillows let you prop up each baby securely so you can sit facing both babies and holding their bottles. These pillows will also come in handy when your twins are learning to sit unassisted. Two bouncer seats can serve this purpose too.

Get twice the recommended number of cloth diapers. You'll use them as burp cloths, bibs, and more. Stash them all over your home, in your diaper bag, and in your car.

Borrow bulky items like bouncer seats and swings. They'll come in handy when you're attempting to appease two babies, but will serve you for only a few months. If you can't borrow them, buy one before committing to a second—a bouncer seat may calm one baby while only a swing will do the trick with the other.

Except for pacifiers, C-shaped pillows, bouncer seats, and favorite toys, do not buy two of everything. Your twins can easily fit on one activity mat or under one activity gym.

MEDICINE CABINET

There's no need to double the quantities, with the exception of items that will go into a sick baby's nose or mouth (nasal aspirator, Baby Tylenol, etc.). But do stock up on the basics.

ON THE GO

You'll need an extra-large diaper bag for day trips, a smaller one for short outings. Buy a backpack version to keep both your hands free. Consider infant car seats since your babies are likely to be small and may get lost in a full-size convertible car seat. Definitely get a double stroller so you can motor the twins around single-handedly. Side by side versions allow both babies to look out but may not fit through some doorways. Front/back versions give one baby priority seating but don't have fit issues. Try them out in the store to assess their ease of handling and folding. You may want to buy one or two inexpensive umbrella strollers as well for those times when you're out with one baby alone, but you can decide that later. A soft baby carrier is great for twins: It allows you to carry one while tending to the other. Don't invest in a second carrier until you see how you and your babies like it.

Traveling distances with your babies will be a challenge, so wait before buying portable cribs. If you do travel occasionally, borrow portable cribs from friends or neighbors.

NURSERY PLAN-O-GRAM

This is your tool if...

- *You've bought your baby furniture but aren't sure how it will best fit your nursery.*
- *You're debating between different-sized cribs or dressers because you're not sure how they'll fit in your space.*
- *You can't wait to get the baby's room organized and want to picture what it will look like.*

Follow these simple instructions:

1 Measure your nursery space and draw it out on the grid on the next page. Each square equals six inches; two squares equal one foot. The grid gives you 15 feet across and 18 feet down. Note doors, windows, closets, outlets, heat and air conditioning vents.

2 Measure your furniture and draw each item out on a photocopy of the grid below, using the same scale. Label each piece and cut it out.

3 Place the pieces on your nursery grid and move them around until you find the best layout. Make sure electrical appliances are near outlets and keep the crib away from drafty windows or vents.

Have fun!

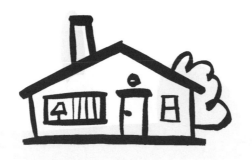

● ● ● COMPARISON SHOPPING

Use these worksheets for pricey items; they'll help you decide which store, catalog, or Web site offers the best option for you.

ITEM:	OPTION 1	OPTION 2	OPTION 3
STORE/CATALOG/WEB SITE			
ADDRESS/PHONE			
CONTACT PERSON			
ITEM DESCRIPTION *(brand, model, color, other)*			
FEATURES			
TIMING/AVAILABILITY			
COST *(price, delivery, set-up, other)*			
ADDITIONAL NOTES			

ITEM:	OPTION 1	OPTION 2	OPTION 3
STORE/CATALOG/WEB SITE			
ADDRESS/PHONE			
CONTACT PERSON			
ITEM DESCRIPTION (brand, model, color, other)			
FEATURES			
TIMING/AVAILABILITY			
COST (price, delivery, set-up, other)			
ADDITIONAL NOTES			

ITEM:	OPTION 1	OPTION 2	OPTION 3
STORE/CATALOG/WEB SITE			
ADDRESS/PHONE			
CONTACT PERSON			
ITEM DESCRIPTION (brand, model, color, other)			
FEATURES			
TIMING/AVAILABILITY			
COST (price, delivery, set-up, other)			
ADDITIONAL NOTES			

• • • BORROWED ITEMS

List items as you borrow them so you remember to return them to their proper owner.

ITEM DESCRIPTION

BORROWED FROM

DUE BACK ON

RETURNED ON

ITEM DESCRIPTION

BORROWED FROM

DUE BACK ON

RETURNED ON

ITEM DESCRIPTION

BORROWED FROM

DUE BACK ON

RETURNED ON

ITEM DESCRIPTION

BORROWED FROM

DUE BACK ON

RETURNED ON

ITEM DESCRIPTION

BORROWED FROM

DUE BACK ON

RETURNED ON

ITEM DESCRIPTION

BORROWED FROM

DUE BACK ON

RETURNED ON

BORROWED ITEMS *(continued)*

ITEM DESCRIPTION

BORROWED FROM

DUE BACK ON

RETURNED ON

ITEM DESCRIPTION

BORROWED FROM

DUE BACK ON

RETURNED ON

ITEM DESCRIPTION

BORROWED FROM

DUE BACK ON

RETURNED ON

ITEM DESCRIPTION

BORROWED FROM

DUE BACK ON

RETURNED ON

ITEM DESCRIPTION

BORROWED FROM

DUE BACK ON

RETURNED ON

ITEM DESCRIPTION

BORROWED FROM

DUE BACK ON

RETURNED ON

BABY SHOWER & GIFTS

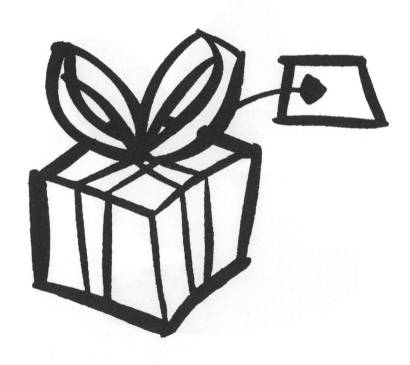

● ● ● REAL MOM TIPS: GIVING THANKS

During your pregnancy and in the months following your baby's arrival,
you're likely to benefit from many kindnesses and gifts. Maybe it was
your sister who listened to your fears and offered encouragement, your
co-workers who threw a surprise shower in your honor, your best friend
who did your laundry and kept you company while you were on bed
rest, or the neighbor who delivered a home-cooked meal the day you got
home from the hospital. And that's not counting the flowers and baby
gifts you received from well-wishers near and far. Whatever the favor or
the present, however large or small, courtesy dictates you acknowledge
such gestures with a written thank-you.

KEEP TRACK

Keep track of gifts and good deeds as soon as you receive them. (A new mom's
memory isn't fail-safe so use the Gifts and Thank-You's log later in this chapter.)
Ideally, you'll want to send out thank-you's as you go, especially before the baby's
birth when you'll have more time. If you let the list grow too long, you may feel
overwhelmed and put off the task altogether. Once your baby is born, you'll be
busy recuperating and caring for your newborn, so take a break from the card
writing. It's perfectly acceptable and understandable to let thank-you's slide a few
months once you're caring full-time for your baby. As long as you jot down gifts
and favors, you'll be in good shape to tackle the task when you're up to it.

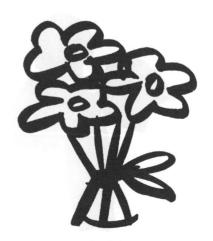

For the most part, a short note is all that's called for, one that speaks from the heart in describing how much the gift or good deed meant to you. You can buy thank-you notes that match your announcements, customized with your baby's name, or buy any off-the-shelf cards. In some cases where an unusual kindness was granted, a token of appreciation in addition to a card is warranted. This need not be elaborate, as the following examples will show.

- Bring a beautiful bouquet of flowers to the hostess of your baby shower; she'll be able to use it as a centerpiece for the refreshment table. Send a thank-you note later recounting favorite moments.

- Treat your best friend to lunch or a pedicure to thank her for her regular visits while you were on bed rest.

- Present a nice bottle of wine to the experienced mom who took you out shopping for baby essentials when you couldn't tackle the project alone.

- Offer pretty coasters or festive candles to the neighbor who bought groceries for you during the last weeks of your pregnancy.

- Give small boxes of specialty chocolates to key nurses and other staff who took such good care of you and your newborn while you were in the hospital.

- Return a maternity wardrobe to its owner, freshly laundered or dry-cleaned, with a note and a gift bag of scented soaps and hand cream.

- Send a fruit basket to the grandparents who spent two weeks with you after the baby's birth, helping with the baby and the household, and giving you and your partner a much-needed break.

These are just a few ideas. Ideally, you'll want to tailor your thank-you gift to the recipient's likes and interests.

● ● ● BABY SHOWER

Jot down details of your baby shower for posterity.

DATE	TIME

GIVEN BY

LOCATION

DETAILS

GUEST LIST

MEMORABLE GIFTS AND SURPRISES

● ● ● GIFTS AND THANK-YOU'S

Keep track of family, friends, and neighbors who send a gift, deliver a meal, lend you something, or run an errand for you. Make sure to note when you sent a thank-you card.

DATE	GIFT/GOOD DEED	FROM	THANKS SENT

● ● ● **GIFTS AND THANK-YOU'S** *(continued)*

DATE	GIFT/GOOD DEED	FROM	THANKS SENT

DATE	GIFT/GOOD DEED	FROM	THANKS SENT

GIFTS AND THANK-YOU'S *(continued)*

DATE	GIFT/GOOD DEED	FROM	THANKS SENT

LABOR & DELIVERY

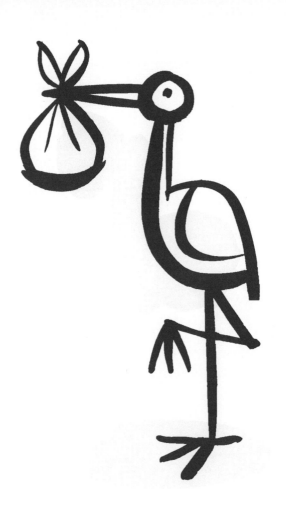

● ● ● REAL MOM TIPS: ENJOYING (GASP!) D-DAY

Ask any parent what their most memorable moment has been to date and the answer is near universal: The birth of their child.

Still, many women are anxious at the thought of experiencing labor and delivery for the first time. You may go through the first and second trimesters basking in the wonder of impending motherhood; but as the delivery date approaches, you realize that this baby will be coming out soon, and that you'll need to take an active role in making that happen.

So, for all you concerned moms-to-be, here's some advice from the delivery room trenches...

DON'T OVERANALYZE

Of course you'll read books, eagerly ask your friends about their experiences, even watch an actual delivery in your childbirth class. You'll hear everything from quick and blissful labors to 30-hour labors followed by emergency c-sections. Remember that each delivery is unique to each woman. Know the basics, then stop—more information may actually increase your anxiety.

Focus on the things that are under your control: Find an OB you trust and a labor coach you can count on, fill out your coach's to-do list and the phone call list, think through your birthing plan, and pack your hospital bag (all in this chapter). Then let nature take its course.

In your last trimester, run through this chapter with your labor coach so that he or she understands your wishes and his or her responsibilities during labor and delivery. When labor does begin in earnest, you'll be able to relinquish control. Stay calm, focus on your experience, and be sure to communicate your needs to your coach.

EXPECT SURPRISES

You may have a concept of how the whole labor and delivery experience will play out; you may even have imagined it step by step, based on what you've read and heard. Again, each woman's experience is very individual. You are likely to be surprised along the way and need to be prepared for things not going exactly as planned. You won't really understand your feelings and needs until you get into the delivery room.

Give yourself permission to change your mind and alter your birthing plan as you go. Whether you're in more pain than you thought and now wish to receive an epidural, or you can't stand your coach touching you during contractions, speak up! Also, remember that your OB is the best judge of what treatment is needed for you and your baby's well-being. You may be overdue and need to be induced, or may have a breech baby and need a c-section. When it comes to your medical care, put your trust in your doctor and his staff.

For a few of you, the labor and delivery experience may turn out to be unexpectedly difficult, maybe because of complications with you or with the baby. Or the whole thing may be a letdown, whether because you had an undesired c-section or you didn't feel a rush of love for your new baby. If you feel "robbed" of the labor and delivery experience, allow yourself to grieve; your regret should dissipate over time, as you fall in love with your baby. If not, get help: Ask your OB or your friends for counselor recommendations (and see organizations that can help in the RESOURCES chapter of this book).

Remember, there is no *right* way to have a baby.

ENJOY THIS AMAZING EXPERIENCE

For most of you, delivering your baby will be an unbelievable experience, even if it's stressful and painful at times. You'll only go through this "first" once in your life, so savor it: Notice your surroundings, remember your nurses' faces and words of encouragement, share your emotions with your coach. Whatever discomfort you may feel will become a distant memory compared to the elation of meeting your son or daughter for the very first time. As soon as you can, write it all down for posterity: Your child will love reading the account of his or her birth many years from now, when details have long faded from your memory.

● ● ● COACH'S TO-DO LIST

When you suspect you are in labor, contact your coach and have him/her run through this checklist.

> **COACH'S NAME AND PHONE**

> **ALTERNATE COACH'S NAME AND PHONE**

First things first:

- Call the OB's office.

> **OBSTETRICIAN NAME AND PHONE**

- Time contractions and note them on the Tracking Your Labor chart.
- Make sure the hospital bag is ready—see the Packing Your Hospital Bag checklist.
- Make necessary phone calls—see the Phone Calls list.
  - for help with older children, animals, or household responsibilities
  - to doulas or others who will be at the birth
- Follow the doctor's orders: ....

....

....

....

....

....

....

....

When given the go-ahead by the OB, head to the hospital:

TAXI COMPANY NAME AND PHONE

Directions/Entrance (including after hours):

Parking/Special instructions:

Once at the hospital, during labor and delivery:

Handle any last-minute paperwork.

Request a private room for post-delivery (if it doesn't come standard and you're willing to pay the upcharge).

Make the mom-to-be comfortable with pillows, music, magazines, candles, whatever she needs.

Make any necessary phone calls to alert family, work, or others—see the Phone Calls list.

Assist the mom-to-be in communicating her Birthing Plan to the nurses and doctors on site, if needed.

Coach her through contractions.

Other instructions:

After the birth:

- Help the new mom settle into her hospital room.
- If she's in pain, ask about pain management medications.
- Assist the new mom in communicating preferences for baby's care to the nurses.
- Make sure the pediatrician's office has been notified to come examine the baby.

> PEDIATRICIAN NAME AND PHONE

- Make phone calls with the joyous news—see the Phone Calls list.
- Learn as much as you can from the nurses about caring for baby— ask questions!
- If mom is planning to nurse, ask to see the lactation consultant on staff.
- Fill out birth certificate and social security information.
- Buy (or have others buy) favorite newspapers and magazines—their front pages or covers make great keepsakes for baby's album.
- Jot down all flowers and presents received at the hospital—see the Gift and Thank-You's log.
- Call in baby information for custom-printed birth announcements (see the BACK HOME chapter).
- Arrange for pick-up or delivery of a reserved breast pump.

> STORE NAME AND PHONE

- Write out thank-you notes to hospital staff who were particularly helpful so you can hand them out with a little treat when you leave.
- Take pictures!
- Other instructions:

Before leaving the hospital:

- Pack up all bags, including free hospital supplies and breast pump attachments, if available.
- Help mom and baby get ready to go home.
- Remember to take flowers and other gifts home (you could even take care of this on a previous trip home, so you can be free to concentrate on mom and baby at this time).
- Make sure you have all necessary prescriptions and special instructions for mom and baby, as well as phone numbers for breastfeeding consultants and other specialists.
- Make a point to thank all hospital staff who took care of mom and baby. Hand out any treats and thank-you notes you may have brought with you at this time.
- Pull up the car with a securely installed infant car seat and a head support for baby's unsteady head.
- Other instructions:

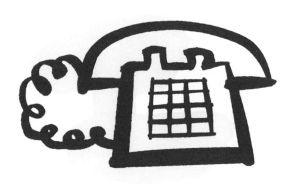

● ● ● **PHONE CALLS**

Prioritize your calls for easy dialing when the time comes.

CALLS TO MAKE WHILE IN LABOR AT HOME:

CALLS TO MAKE WHILE IN LABOR AT THE HOSPITAL:

CALLS TO MAKE AFTER THE BABY IS BORN:

CALLS TO MAKE BEFORE HEADING HOME:

CALLS TO MAKE ONCE BACK AT HOME:

● ● ● TRACKING YOUR LABOR

Your obstetrician will ask how far apart your contractions are: This means the minutes from the start of one contraction to the start of the next. This chart will help you time your contractions and determine if they are getting closer together. Jot down the time at which each contraction started, the interval between the start of one contraction and the start of the next, and notes such as the degree and location of pain, signs of bleeding or leaking fluid, etc.

START TIME	INTERVAL	NOTES

START TIME	INTERVAL	NOTES

● ● ● PACKING YOUR HOSPITAL BAG

FOR LABOR AND DELIVERY

- [ ] Cash for a taxi ride to the hospital, just in case
- [ ] Hospital preregistration information
- [ ] Insurance card/information
- [ ] Eyeglasses/contact lens case/solution
- [ ] Calling card or change (if needed for phone calls and vending machines)
- [ ] Reading, videotapes, games, etc.
- [ ] Hair band (to tie back long hair)
- [ ] Lotion (for dry skin and coach's massages)
- [ ] Lip balm (to keep lips moist)
- [ ] Comfortable old pillow(s) and pillowcase(s)
- [ ] Heavy socks (to keep feet warm)
- [ ] Portable CD or tape player with music
- [ ] Camera with extra film and fresh batteries
- [ ] Video camera with extra tape and battery
- [ ] Snacks and beverages (for coach during labor)
- [ ] Snacks and beverages (for mom after delivery)
- [ ] This book

FOR MOM IN HER HOSPITAL ROOM

- [ ] Toiletries and hair dryer
- [ ] Maternity panties
- [ ] Doughnut to sit on (hospital may provide)
- [ ] Nursing bras and pads
- [ ] Nightgowns or nursing gowns

- ( ) Robe or soft cardigan
- ( ) Nonskid slippers
- ( ) Make-up (if desired)
- ( ) Loose going-home clothes and comfortable shoes
- ( )
- ( )
- ( )

FOR LABOR COACH

- ( ) Toiletries, change of clothes
- ( ) Cash, calling card, keys, etc.
- ( ) Prioritized list of whom to call (like the Phone Calls list earlier in this chapter)
- ( )
- ( )
- ( )

FOR BABY

- ( ) Receiving blankets
- ( ) Burp cloths
- ( ) Going home outfit appropriate to the weather
- ( ) Diaper bag with newborn diapers, wipes, change of clothes, bottles, pacifier
- ( ) Car seat with head support
- ( )
- ( )
- ( )

FOR HOSPITAL STAFF (AS DESIRED)

- ( ) Thank-you cards to fill out and distribute before leaving
- ( ) Small gifts such as little boxes of chocolates or scented soaps to hand out with the cards
- ( )
- ( )
- ( )

● ● ● BIRTHING PLAN

Discuss your preferences with your obstetrician and labor coach in person, before the birth. Just be aware that a turn of events could necessitate a change of plans.

I PREFER TO LABOR... *(where, in what position, with whom, etc.)*

MY VIEW ON PAIN MEDICATION IS...

I WOULD LIKE TO BE MADE COMFORTABLE WITH... *(music, lighting, massage, ice chips, shower, etc.)*

I PREFER TO DELIVER... *(position, use of mirror, draping, episiotomy, photos, etc.)*

WHEN MY BABY IS BORN, I WOULD LIKE... *(cutting cord, nursing baby, photos, etc.)*

....

....

....

....

WHEN IT COMES TO THE CARE OF MY BABY, I PREFER... *(rooming in, nursing, formula, pacifiers, circumcision, etc.)*

....

....

....

....

DURING RECOVERY IN MY HOSPITAL ROOM, I WOULD LIKE... *(visitors, calls, bathing, food, medication etc.)*

....

....

....

....

● ● ● MEETING BABY

BABY'S NAME

| DATE OF BIRTH | TIME OF BIRTH | WEIGHT | LENGTH |

TEST RESULTS:

DISTINGUISHING MARKS:

FIRST IMPRESSIONS:

● ● ● INSTRUCTIONS FOR MOM AND BABY CARE

Jot down recommendations from your doctors and nurses to help you recover at home and to attend to your newborn's needs.

TAKING CARE OF MOM:

TAKING CARE OF BABY:

BACK HOME

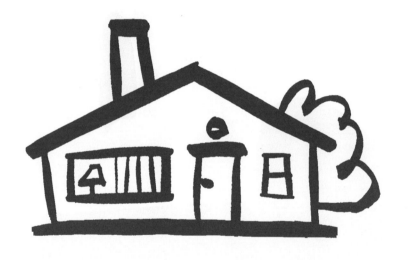

The first months with a new baby will have their highs and lows. While you're still marveling at this little creature, so perfect in every tiny detail, you're bound to experience some difficulties adjusting to life with a newborn.

You're sore and sleep deprived, you're nervous about your new role as a mom, you're worried about your newborn's health, you're frustrated with nursing, you're cooped up at home, you're not bonding with baby, you're inundated with visitors, you're fighting with your partner... These are just a few of the feelings you may encounter at home with your newborn...and you're not alone.

For help in surviving those first months, take these hints from new moms to heart.

REDUCE YOUR EXPECTATIONS

You may have anticipated weeks of blissful bonding with your new baby, snuggling up together for catnaps, nursing with ease while your partner looks on lovingly. This picture of perfect family harmony and unity may not materialize just as you envisioned it. Your role as a parent will develop over time and with experience. For now, don't expect too much of yourself. You've just been through a physical feat and need time and rest to recover.

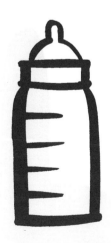

Do the minimum. Have your baby sleep next to your bed in a bassinet to reduce ups and downs, particularly at night. Nap when your newborn naps. Turn off the phone's ringer and let the answering machine pick up messages. Discourage visits from anyone who's not willing to provide a helping hand or who expects to be entertained. Make it ok to stay in your pj's all day and let the house get messy. Take a long, hot bath and listen to soothing music when you're not napping. Order in or eat frozen meals. Your primary job is to take care of yourself and your baby.

If your life seems hopelessly out of control and you get a headache just thinking about your to-do list, take small steps to reduce the chaos. Set manageable goals, like returning one phone call or writing one thank-you note each day.

WELCOME OFFERS OF HELP

Your family and friends will probably be eager to help, so let them. Do you need groceries purchased? Laundry washed? Announcement envelopes stuffed? A prescription picked up? A home-cooked meal? Make your wishes known. Consider asking your mom, sister, or a friend to stay with you the first week or two and lend an experienced hand. It's also not too late to call baby nurses: They may have had a cancellation and be able to give you a night off, even just once a week.

Seek out experts to deal with a particular issue. Baby not latching on? Call your hospital's lactation consultant. Feeling blue? Talk to your OB; she can direct you to a counselor if she suspects depression (see the RESOURCES chapter, too). So sleep-deprived you can't see straight? Ask your partner to take over a few night feedings with pumped breast milk or formula.

Don't forget to write down who has done what for you (see the BABY SHOWERS AND GIFTS chapter). When the fog of the first weeks clears, you'll want to remember helpful gestures with a thank-you note.

GET OUT OF THE HOUSE

After a few weeks, once you're feeling better and starting to get the hang of this mommy thing, venture out with your newborn for some fresh air, even for just a brief stroll around the neighborhood. Most babies are incredibly portable during their first few months, before they settle into a routine. Take advantage of this and gradu- ate to longer excursions to the mall, park, or grocery store. Meet a friend for lunch, set up a regular "playdate" with a neighbor, join a new moms' group. Don't forget to bring a stocked diaper bag with all of baby's needs, just in case (see Packing the Diaper Bag in this chapter). And once in a while, seek out personal, adult time. Ask a family member or your partner to watch the baby while you get out of the house: There's nothing like a pedicure or a coffee with a friend to lift your spirits.

DON'T NEGLECT YOUR PARTNER

In the joy and exhaustion of recovering from delivery and caring for a newborn, you're likely to focus less on your relationship. Your partner may be going through adjustments of his own: He may be unsure of his role as a father, may feel awkward handling the baby, may even grow resentful as he watches you fall in love with the newest family member. The two of you may struggle with how to divide up baby and household responsibilities.

Because you'll probably be the primary caregiver for your newborn, you'll be able to read your baby's needs and respond to them faster and better than anyone else. Don't expect your partner to meet your standards. Do encourage his involvement with the baby's care and allow him to develop his own rituals with baby; in short, give him an opportunity to bond too. Ideally, allow him some time alone with baby, away from your watchful eye—this will give you a break too!

Make sure your partner knows how important he is to you and to the family. Small gestures will go a long way: A snuggle, a conversation about his day, a ques- tion about his feelings. When you're up to it, enlist grandparents to babysit for a few hours so you can enjoy a dinner out solo with your partner (try to spend at least part of the time talking about something other than your bundle of joy). Discuss concerns as they arise, before resentment turns into anger, and seek out a mutually acceptable solution. Remember, a strong relationship between you and your partner is the essential foundation of a happy family.

● ● ● FEEDING AND DIAPERING

Make sure your baby is feeding enough, as well as wetting diapers regularly, by filling out this chart. Jot down the time of each feeding, how much baby ate (minutes if you're nursing; ounces if you're bottle-feeding), a wet or soiled diaper, and other notes such as which side you nursed on or the occurrence of a loose stool. Call your pediatrician with questions or concerns and bring this information to your baby's next checkup. This log will also come in handy if you're sharing baby care responsibilities with your partner or a caregiver. After several months, you may start to see patterns develop, in which case you can anticipate your baby's needs and start settling into a schedule.

TIME	AMOUNT	WET/SOILED	NOTES	DATE:

TIME	AMOUNT	WET/SOILED	NOTES	DATE:

TIME	AMOUNT	WET/SOILED	NOTES	DATE:

● ● ● PACKING THE DIAPER BAG

When leaving the house, pack these essentials so you're always ready to meet your baby's changing needs.

- Changing pad
- Diapers
- Wipes in travel case (or in plastic storage bag)
- Plastic bag for wet or soiled diapers
- Diaper rash ointment
- Hand wipes or sanitizer
- Tissue
- If nursing: Privacy blanket, change of shirt or sweater/jacket, extra nursing pads
- If bottle-feeding: Pre-measured bottles of water and travel formula container or empty bottles with single-serve cans of formula
- Baby food and spoon (for an older baby)
- Snacks (for you or an older baby)
- Bibs
- Burp cloths or cloth diapers
- Change of baby clothes, hat and outerwear if it turns cold, wide-brimmed hat if it turns sunny
- Blanket
- Pacifier or other security object (if using)
- Rattles and other small toys
- Medications (as needed)

● ○ ◦ CELEBRATING THE BIRTH

A religious ceremony or other celebration calls for some planning. Let this log help you maintain critical information.

OCCASION	DATE
LOCATION	TIME

PLANNING NOTES:

GUEST LIST:

● ● ● CUSTOM ANNOUNCEMENTS

Keep all your information regarding custom announcements in one place.

STATIONER OR SUPPLIER

CONTACT NAME	PHONE	FAX

ANNOUNCEMENT ORDER DETAILS:

WORDING OF ANNOUNCEMENT:

DATE ORDERED ANNOUNCEMENTS AND
ENVELOPES, MATCHING THANK-YOU CARDS:

DATE EXPECT TO RECEIVE ENVELOPES IF
WILL ADDRESS BEFORE THE BIRTH:

INSTRUCTIONS TO CALL IN BABY INFORMATION AT BIRTH:

● ● ● ANNOUNCEMENT MAILING LIST

Go through your address book to decide to whom you'll send announcements. Put the recipients' names below and check them off once you've mailed their announcements. Or, use this space as a reminder to send birth announcements to your OB, pediatrician, doula, and other professionals. They will certainly appreciate a memento of the birth and may even display photos of new arrivals in their offices.

○ _____   ○ _____

○ _____   ○ _____

○ _____   ○ _____

○ _____   ○ _____

○ _____   ○ _____

○ _____   ○ _____

○ _____   ○ _____

○ _____   ○ _____

○ _____   ○ _____

○ _____   ○ _____

○ _____   ○ _____

○ _____   ○ _____

○ _____   ○ _____

○ _____   ○ _____

○ _____   ○ _____

HEALTHCARE FOR BABY

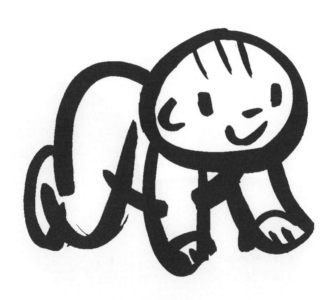

● ● ● REAL MOM TIPS: TEAMING UP WITH YOUR PEDIATRICIAN

Your pediatrician will be an important resource for you, particularly in the early years of your child's life. It pays to research your options carefully and to develop a good working relationship with the doctor of your choice.

Gather recommendations from doctors and like-minded parents (jot them down on the Potential Pediatricians form), speak to the office staff to make sure your basic requirements are met (see below), then ask to interview the doctor. Ideally, you'll want to interview the pediatrician in person, with your partner, and before the baby's birth (see the Interview form). It's well worth it, even for a nominal fee. The interview will also provide an opportunity to check out the office and meet the staff.

Keep in mind the following tips in choosing a pediatrician.

BASIC REQUIREMENTS

Call the office and speak to a staff person in charge. Make sure the following basics meet your needs before requesting an interview with the pediatrician.

1 **Insurance:** The practice should be covered by your insurance plan and accepting new patients. Ideally, they'll process claims directly with your insurance company and have a billing specialist you can contact with questions.

2 **Certification and affiliation:** Pediatricians in the practice should be board-certified by the American Board of Pediatrics, state-licensed, and affiliated with a reputable children's hospital. Your pediatrician should have privileges at the hospital where you'll deliver so he/she can examine your newborn the day of delivery.

3 **Location:** Expect frequent visits to your pediatrician. Look for a practice that's close to your home and has plenty of convenient parking, especially helpful when you're maneuvering a sick child, car seat or stroller, and diaper bag.

4 **Hours:** Look for evening and weekend hours, particularly if you work outside the home. Find out how much time the office will allot for a well-child visit, and how quickly you can get in to see the doctor with a sick child. Ideally, the practice should have a daily drop-in hour for sudden illnesses and a call-in hour for minor questions.

5 **Size:** A large practice may offer better hours and more on-site services (such as x-rays and lab testing) but may be more impersonal and may decrease the chance that you'll visit with your baby's primary doctor when you come in unexpectedly. You should feel comfortable with all the doctors in the practice, even if you prefer your own.

6 **Responsiveness:** Make sure you're able to reach a pediatrician in your practice 24 hours a day with an emergency, and understand how long it will take for a doctor or nurse to call you back on minor matters. Also, assess how easy it is to get through to the office on the phone, and ask how long you should expect to be in the waiting room when you're in for a scheduled appointment.

7 **Other:** The office should be clean and neat, the staff knowledgeable and friendly.

As a new mother, you'll probably have many questions and need direction on anything from putting baby on a schedule to taking a rectal temperature. Make sure your pediatrician is willing to take the time to listen to your concerns, show genuine interest in your child, and coach you on your baby's care and development. Observe the doctor's bedside manner with your child: Does he/she handle your baby gently, call your baby by name, and recall your baby's history?

Look for a pediatrician who shares, or at least supports, your views on controversial issues such as nursing, sleep, circumcision, or pacifiers. Is your doctor a parent? Make sure he or she provides realistic instructions for your baby's care.

Ideally, you'll want to establish a solid long-term relationship with your pediatrician. Follow these tips to foster a bond with your doctor.

1 **Read, read, read.** Invest in a few good books on baby care and development; subscribe to magazines so you're updated on topical issues (see the RESOURCES chapter). Talk to your mom-friends. Be prepared for a fruitful discussion with your pediatrician, and make an educated decision together.

2 **Maintain your baby's records.** You should be the keeper of your baby's health information, including measurements, immunizations, conditions, illnesses, operations, allergies, and reactions to medications (see Baby's Health Log and Growth Chart in this chapter).

3 **Be prepared.** Bring your Baby's Health log and Growth Chart and your questions to every visit. When calling or visiting your doctor due to an illness, have detailed notes handy (see Pediatrician Calls).

4 **Respect your pediatrician's time.** Reserve late night and weekend calls for urgent matters. Call the office during regular hours with routine questions or save them for your next doctor visit (note them on your Pediatrician Visit form).

It's also important that you build a relationship with your pediatrician's staff. Receptionists can make sure you receive prompt service, billing specialists can follow up on insurance issues for you, and pediatric nurses will often handle your baby's shots and your routine questions. Greet them by name, treat them with respect, and thank them for their efforts on your behalf.

Remember that it takes time to build a rapport with a new doctor. Don't compromise on your child's well-being but be willing to work out minor disagreements. If you don't feel you can be candid with issues you have about your doctor or the practice, or if your concerns are not addressed to your satisfaction, it's time to leave. Find out from your insurance carrier how to make the switch, sign up with a new pediatrician, and then call the old practice to have your baby's records transferred. As a courtesy, call your pediatrician to explain your departure, hopefully prompting change in that practice.

• ◦ ● POTENTIAL PEDIATRICIANS

NAME   PHONE

RECOMMENDED BY

NOTES

NAME   PHONE

RECOMMENDED BY

NOTES

NAME   PHONE

RECOMMENDED BY

NOTES

● ○ ● PEDIATRICIAN INTERVIEW

Come early to the interview so you can check out the office (Is it conve-
nient, inviting, clean? Are there toys?), the staff (Are they pleasant?
Professional?), even chat with other parents in the waiting room (What
do they like and dislike about the practice? About each doctor?). If
you were unclear about the office staff responses to some of the "basic
requirement" questions outlined at the beginning of the chapter, feel
free to discuss them further with the pediatrician. Otherwise, stick to
more substantive questions such as the ones outlined below.

BACKGROUND

- What is your education and training? Are you state-licensed and board-certified?
- How many years have you been in practice? What about the other doctors in your group?
- When are you in the office? Will I always see a doctor (as opposed to a nurse or physician assistant) when I come to the office? What is the "on call" schedule when the office is closed?
- How are referrals to specialists handled? Prescription refills? How quickly are they handled?

PHILOSOPHY

- What is your philosophy of care?
- How do you feel about…(issues of concern to you such as breastfeeding, pacifiers, co-sleeping, circumcision, establishing a schedule, use of antibiotics)?
- Do you do all aspects of each exam? Do you explain each part of the exam as it's being performed? Do you set time aside for a discussion of baby's progress? Do you give written instructions on the baby's care? How do you handle developmental concerns?

CHECKUPS

- Will you come to the hospital to examine my baby soon after the birth? Who will notify you?

- When will I bring my baby to your office for a first checkup? Will you provide me with a schedule of well-baby appointments? How long will you typically spend with us at these appointments?
- What first aid/medicine items should I have on hand?
- What do you expect from parents?

THE NEXT STEP

- How do I sign on with you?

NOTES

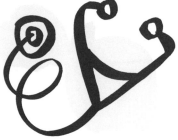

• ● • PEDIATRICIAN BASICS

PRIMARY PEDIATRICIAN'S NAME

OTHER DOCTORS IN THE PRACTICE

OTHER STAFF IN THE PRACTICE

MAIN PHONE NUMBER

OTHER NUMBERS

ADDRESS/DIRECTIONS/PARKING

OFFICE HOURS

EMERGENCY PROCEDURE/OTHER INSTRUCTIONS

BABY'S HEALTH INSURANCE BASICS

HEALTH INSURANCE PLAN

TYPE OF PLAN

PRIMARY MEMBER

MEMBER SOCIAL SECURITY NUMBER

GROUP NUMBER

ID NUMBER

PHONE NUMBER

OTHER NUMBERS

ADDRESS TO SEND CLAIMS TO

OTHER

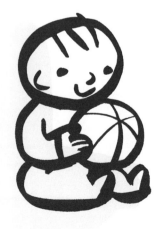

● ● ● BABY'S HEALTH

| DATE OF BIRTH | BLOOD TYPE | SOCIAL SECURITY NUMBER |

CONDITIONS AND ALLERGIES

DATE	TYPE	NOTES

MEDICATIONS

DATE	TYPE	NOTES

DATE	TYPE	NOTES

ILLNESSES, INJURIES, AND SURGERIES

DATE	TYPE	NOTES

BABY'S GROWTH CHART

DATE	WEIGHT	LENGTH	HEAD CIRCUMFERENCE

● ● ● PEDIATRICIAN VISITS

Bring a diaper bag stocked with all the essentials, including extra bottles, snacks, and toys for unexpected waits. Dress your baby in clothing that's easy to put on and take off. A blanket comes in handy if you've undressed your baby in a cold exam room. Come ready with questions!

DATE   TIME   DOCTOR

QUESTIONS TO ASK

NOTES/INSTRUCTIONS

DATE   TIME   DOCTOR

QUESTIONS TO ASK

NOTES/INSTRUCTIONS

DATE   TIME

DOCTOR

QUESTIONS TO ASK

NOTES/INSTRUCTIONS

DATE   TIME

DOCTOR

QUESTIONS TO ASK

NOTES/INSTRUCTIONS

● ● ● PEDIATRICIAN CALLS

When calling due to illness, be prepared. Remind the doctor of your child's name and age, health conditions and medical problems, medications, and allergies. Describe your baby's symptoms (including mood and appetite), when they started and how they've changed over time, rectal temperature readings, treatments you've tried, and your baby's reactions. Have your baby nearby in case the doctor asks you a question that requires an observation or wants to listen to your baby's cough. Be ready to jot down instructions and to give out your pharmacy's phone number.

DATE

DOCTOR/NURSE

QUESTIONS TO ASK

NOTES/INSTRUCTIONS

DATE

DOCTOR/NURSE

QUESTIONS TO ASK

NOTES/INSTRUCTIONS

DATE

DOCTOR/NURSE

QUESTIONS TO ASK

NOTES/INSTRUCTIONS

DATE

DOCTOR/NURSE

QUESTIONS TO ASK

NOTES/INSTRUCTIONS

DATE

DOCTOR/NURSE

QUESTIONS TO ASK

NOTES/INSTRUCTIONS

● INSURANCE RECORDS

Stay on top of medical expenses by tracking payments made by you or your insurance carrier for all pediatric services.

DATE OF SERVICE	PROVIDER	DESCRIPTION OF SERVICE	FEE	CO-PAY	INSURANCE PAYMENT	BALANCE DUE	PAYMENT MADE

● ● ● INSURANCE CALL LOG

Record dates, names, agreements, and next steps from billing-related conversations with your insurance carrier and pediatric providers.

● ● ● EMERGENCY INFORMATION

Post this list next to every phone in your home along with the Baby's Health log. Remember to update it as needed.

AMBULANCE		POISON CONTROL	
POLICE		FIRE	

PARENT/FAMILY/CAREGIVER PHONE NUMBERS

PEDIATRICIAN   24-HOUR PHARMACY

PARENT/CAREGIVER DOCTORS

NEARBY FRIENDS' PHONE NUMBERS

DIRECTIONS TO NEAREST HOSPITAL *(covered by insurance plan)*

TAXI PHONE NUMBERS

HOME ADDRESS   HOME PHONE

DIRECTIONS TO HOME

See Baby's Health log for vital medical information

● ● ● MEDICAL TREATMENT AUTHORIZATION

In your absence, make sure you leave a copy of this form and a copy of your baby's health insurance card with your child's caregiver.

We, the undersigned parents of:

hereby authorize:

CAREGIVERS

DOCTORS

OTHERS

to act in our behalf to consent to all necessary and appropriate medical treatment, surgery, or hospital care, which is advisable by, and to be rendered under the general care of, a licensed physician or surgeon under the laws of the state of

MOTHER'S SIGNATURE   FATHER'S SIGNATURE

DATE   DATE

ADDRESS

PHONE NUMBERS

MEDICAL INSURANCE

CHILDCARE

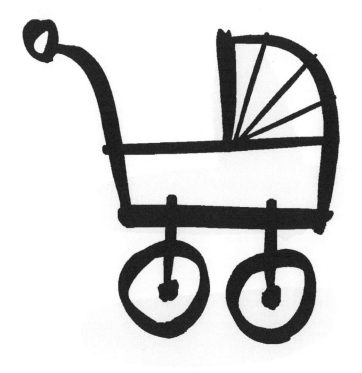

● ● ● REAL MOM TIPS: FINDING GREAT CHILDCARE

Unless you're lucky enough to have family willing and able to help care for your baby, you'll need to look for childcare at some point in the first year. Most of us are busy with jobs or activities outside the home and, in any case, we all need a break once in a while. Looking for childcare can be a nerve-wracking and tedious process, although finding the right caregiver is ultimately a rewarding experience.

Ideally, you'll want to interview several candidates before making up your mind, so you have a basis for comparison; but don't be afraid to move quickly if you find the perfect caregiver or the ideal daycare. Involve your partner in the quest for childcare, and certainly in the ultimate decision: Two concerned heads are better than one.

Here are tips—based on input from dozens of moms—on how to find great in-home caregivers and daycare facilities, step by step.

STEP 1: ASSESS YOUR NEEDS

An in-home caregiver will provide more flexibility and one-on-one stimulation but is more expensive and offers no back-up if she's ill. Daycare is more reliable and affordable, but offers less personal attention and requires shuttling your baby back and forth. Which is for you?

Turn to experienced moms for points of view on your many options, take a look at your budget, discuss the options with your partner, and refer to the RESOURCES chapter for books and websites that can shed more light on the subject. If you're still unsure, you may choose to evaluate both caregiver and daycare options, and perhaps even use a combination of the two. Even so, you'll need to go one step further in detailing your requirements.

If you're considering an in-home caregiver, ask yourself the following:

    Do you prefer live-in or come-and-go? Will you consider an *au pair*?
    How about sharing a nanny with a friend or neighbor?

- How much flexibility do you require with her schedule?
- How much experience is ideal?
- What responsibilities do you expect of her? Will you need her to drive your baby around?
- How important is English fluency?
- What pay and benefits are you willing to offer?
- Will you need help from an agency in handling nanny tax requirements?

If you prefer the daycare option, think through these questions:

- Do you prefer a small home daycare run by a mom (a family daycare) or a larger daycare center?
- What hours/days of availability do you require?
- How much experience and supervision do you expect?
- How far are you willing to drive from your home or work?
- How much can you afford to pay?

Early on in your pregnancy, do some research. Talk to your doctors, neighbors, co-workers, family, and friends about how to find the best care for your baby. Jot down recommended nanny agencies, daycare centers and family daycares, newspapers with childcare ads, as well as local schools, community centers, and churches/synagogues that accept job postings. Don't neglect your employer—many companies provide a place (board, newsletter, email) for job postings or resources to help you find childcare.

In-Home Caregiver

If you're interested in the *au pair* program, look into it early, about 6 months before you'd like her to start. You'll want to use an accredited *au pair* agency that will help you through all the steps (see the RESOURCES chapter).

Otherwise, start interviewing in-home caregivers close to the time when you want them to start. When caregivers are interviewing, they're typically looking for immediate work. Word-of-mouth is a great way to find a nanny or babysitter, especially if it's from like-minded parents, so follow up on promising leads. Be aware, however, that each family has specific needs: A caregiver who is perfect for one family may not be right for another.

When placing an ad or posting a job offering, make sure to specify your requirements—job hours and location, need for car, language proficiency, etc.—to avoid responses from unqualified candidates. Also, scan your local paper for caregivers advertising their availability.

A more expensive solution for the time-constrained is to sign up with one or more nanny agencies (many agencies only charge a fee once they've helped you find someone). The International Nanny Association can refer you to member agencies (see the RESOURCES chapter). Speak to the director of potential agencies and find out how they operate, and particularly how thoroughly they evaluate their candidates. At the very least they should interview the candidate personally, speak to three references, and conduct criminal, motor vehicle, and child abuse background checks. If they can certify the candidate's health, check her credit history, verify her social security number, and provide CPR/First Aid training, that's even better. Make sure you're comfortable with their fees and refund policy, and call the agency's references.

Decide which agencies you prefer and fill out their required forms before your baby's birth—it will be one fewer thing to worry about in the first several weeks at home. Again, be as specific as possible about job requirements to avoid wasting your time.

Be sure to fill out the Job Description form provided in this section before interviewing candidates in order to clearly communicate the job's requirements and compensation package.

Daycare Facilities

Start looking for daycare early (at least six months before you'll need it) because the best ones fill up fast. Call the Childcare Aware hotline or use the Internet to find licensed daycares in your area (see the RESOURCES chapter). Inquire about daycare affiliations through your place of work. Talk to neighbors and scan the local newspapers for home daycare openings. The best daycares will be accredited by the National Association for the Education of Young Children (daycare centers) or the National Association of Family Child Care (family daycares), so contact those organizations as well (see Resources chapter). Your Department of Children and Family Services (DCFS) and Better Business Bureau can make you aware of complaints filed against local daycares.

Call recommended daycares, speak to the director to make sure they meet your basic needs, then have information sent to you. Once you have your list of options, schedule in-person interviews, as well as a tour and observation time.

STEP 3: INTERVIEW PROMISING CANDIDATES

You're bound to be a little nervous when conducting interviews. Every caregiver or daycare could be "it", so while you want to ask the tough questions, you're also selling yourself and your family and setting the tone for what could be a long-term relationship. Of course, unless you're in a bidding war for Mary Poppins or putting your child on the top daycare center's waiting list, you're usually in the driver's seat while choosing your childcare. Let the other person do the talking by asking open-ended questions. Take plenty of notes so you can make comparisons and fill in your partner if he was unable to attend. Most importantly, don't compromise on the safety and nurturing of your child.

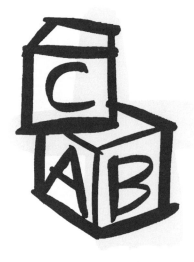

In-Home Caregiver

Once you start getting responses to your ad or recommendations from agencies, be prepared to move quickly—great caregivers get snapped up in no time. First, conduct a quick phone call to screen the candidate, making sure your basic requirements are met and to get an initial reaction to the person. Ask for at least two work and two personal references.

Next, use this section's Reference Interview questionnaire to probe former employers about the candidate. Call the personal references to verify the candidate's information and to see if she'd be a good fit as your child's caregiver. This reference-check process allows you to determine the candidate's strengths and to uncover potential issues you'll want to address in person (check these references even if you're using a nanny agency—you never know how thorough they were or what you can come up with on your own).

Third, assuming you're hearing all the right things, ask the candidate to come to your home for an in-person interview. Ideally, you'll want to talk to the candidate without your baby so you can focus on the discussion and make note of responses, using this section's Caregiver Interview questionnaire. So have a family member or friend watch your baby in another part of your home for a half hour or so. Once you're satisfied the candidate has real potential, introduce her to your baby and watch them interact. Consider scheduling a second interview if you have more questions, your partner could not be there the first time, or you simply need more time with her to be absolutely sure. Above all, trust your instincts. If something doesn't feel quite right, even if you can't put your finger on it, err on the safe side and walk away.

Fourth, offer your chosen candidate the job, discussing schedule, responsibilities, pay, and benefits. Be fair, but be prepared for negotiation, especially on compensation: Have a maximum amount set before this discussion. If you feel unsure, tell the caregiver you need to think about it and get back to her. Always make the offer pending a background check, TB screening, and trial period, as discussed below.

Fifth, conduct a background check on the candidate covering her criminal, motor vehicle, credit, and child abuse history in every state where she has resided, as well as checking her social security information. Many nanny agencies include those in their fee, or you'll want to contact an accredited company to perform the check for you (see the RESOURCES chapter). In that case, you will need to get a signed authorization from the nanny (if she won't sign, walk away). You should pay for your caregiver to undergo a physical and take an Infant CPR/First Aid class (ideally in her native language) before she starts. Make sure the physical includes a screening for tuberculosis (TB), a serious, highly contagious disease with no available vaccine.

Finally, even if your caregiver has cleared all hurdles, try her out for a day when you'll be home. If all goes well, you may still wish to agree on a trial period, from a few days to a month, within which time either party can terminate the relationship. You may also want to put your work agreement in writing and have both of you sign it. Such a document should include employer and employee names and addresses, schedule, pay and benefits, childcare and household rules and responsibilities, as well as a statement on how to terminate the agreement. The more clearly you spell everything out, the better you'll avoid surprises and disagreements later on. Any subsequent changes to a written agreement should be made in writing as well.

Daycare Facilities

It's essential you visit potential daycare facilities to interview the director and caregivers personally, tour the premises, and observe the children and staff in action. Use the Daycare Interview questionnaire as your guide for the director's interview and take lots of notes for future reference. Also, ask to interview the primary caregiver for your baby (use the Caregiver Interview questionnaire as a guide). While you may need to schedule the interviews and tours during naptime so you can receive undivided attention, plan another leisurely observation outside of naptimes, preferably in the afternoon. This will provide a better reflection of the level of personal attention, energy, and patience you can expect for your baby toward the end of a long day.

During the interviews, ask to see samples of written records for infants (including feeding, sleeping, and diaper change logs), the daycare's activity schedules, weekly menus, and policies. But don't just take their word for it. Make sure you visit the food preparation, diaper changing, and sleeping areas, as well as the bathrooms. Ask the director to point things out during the tour, such as emergency information postings, childproofing measures, and diaper disposal.

Ask for references before leaving and call these parents to probe on their experience with the daycare and other daycares they may have looked into or tried out. You may also want to check out a few references for the director. Again, trust your instincts and shy away from any daycare that doesn't feel right. If you've found a great daycare but they can't take your child right away, get onto their waiting list and opt for your second choice on a temporary basis (ask your first choice for recommendations).

STEP 4: MANAGE YOUR CHILDCARE

It's not enough to find and hire great childcare. You'll need to build a strong relationship with your caregiver, whether in-home or at a daycare, to ensure your child gets the best care. Openly discuss concerns that come up and always act with the intent of improving the situation; if you're still not happy, or you feel your baby's well-being is in jeopardy, terminate the relationship and look elsewhere. Nothing is worth compromising your baby's health and safety.

In-Home Caregiver

Allow a brief period of adjustment for your caregiver to get to know your child and fit into your family and routine. Ask her to fill out a daily journal of activities and observations about your child and check up on her with surprise visits. Ideally, your caregiver will become an essential part of your household; you may even come to think of her as family. Treat her as such and she and your child will both benefit from their mutual affection. So ask for her advice and include her in day-to-day activities, provide her the tools for special projects and encourage her ideas, give her freedom while setting guidelines, buy her favorite foods and beverages, praise her often, and don't overwork her or demean her. Reward her efforts with a yearly raise, bonus, extra days off, birthday and holiday gifts, or other perks and privileges. Combat loneliness by introducing her to neighborhood caregivers or signing her up for baby classes. Above all, foster an atmosphere of open communication so issues that arise on either side are discussed and resolved quickly, before they have a chance to turn into bigger problems. Set aside a regular time each week to share views on child-rearing, discuss your child's progress, voice concerns on either side, and go over the family schedule for the next few weeks.

Do come up with a back-up plan for the days when your caregiver may call in sick, whether it's a relative who can fill in for a day or two, a neighbor willing to lend a hand, or a nanny agency with experienced temporary sitters.

Daycare Facilities

Before your baby's first day, meet with the daycare's director and your baby's primary caregiver (one and the same in most family daycares) to go over expectations on both sides as well as how to phase your baby into the program. Ask for their advice and start developing solid relationships. Take this opportunity to discuss your baby's personality and needs and to agree on how you will communicate regularly about progress and issues.

The first week, you may wish to spend part of each day at the daycare with your baby to allow transition time for the both of you. After that, drop in unexpectedly to check up on your baby; get to know the other infants' parents so you can check on each other's children when you're there. Greet all of your baby's caregivers by name, stop and talk to them, ask questions, seek their advice, raise issues promptly, and show your appreciation. Make all payments on time and abide by daycare rules. Attend parents' meetings and teacher conferences to demonstrate your interest and commitment.

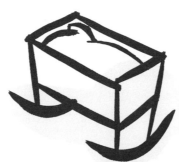

POTENTIAL CAREGIVERS OR DAYCARE FACILITIES

NAME   PHONE

RECOMMENDED BY

NOTES/PHONE CALL LOG

NAME   PHONE

RECOMMENDED BY

NOTES/PHONE CALL LOG

NAME   PHONE

RECOMMENDED BY

NOTES/PHONE CALL LOG

NAME   PHONE

RECOMMENDED BY

NOTES/PHONE CALL LOG

NAME   PHONE

RECOMMENDED BY

NOTES/PHONE CALL LOG

NAME   PHONE

RECOMMENDED BY

NOTES/PHONE CALL LOG

● ● ● CAREGIVER JOB DESCRIPTION

Define the job clearly and there'll be less room for disagreement later on. Alter and refine this as needed, at least once a year.

STARTING DATE	SCHEDULE *(regular, expected overtime)*

CHILDREN'S NAMES, AGES, SPECIAL NEEDS:

PARENTS' SCHEDULES:

CHILDCARE

RESPONSIBILITIES AND PHILOSOPHY:

RULES: *(sweets, TV, discipline, etc.)*

RESPONSIBILITIES:

....

....

RULES: *(TV and phone use, visitors, smoking, safety, petty cash fund, personal errands, etc.)*

....

....

....

FOR IN-HOME CAREGIVERS

LIVING QUARTERS:

....

MORE RULES: *(privacy, eating and travel with the family, maintaining living quarters, curfews, overnight guests, use of car, phone, laundry, kitchen, TV, alcohol, etc.)*

....

....

....

....

COMPENSATION

PAY: *(amount, payday, form of pay, tardiness, performance-based raises, overtime rates, taxes)*

....

BENEFITS: *(vacation, paid holidays, sick days, bonus, car/laundry privileges, auto/health insurance)*

....

....

CAREGIVER REFERENCE INTERVIEW

Always check a candidate's references; you'll often find these conversations very enlightening. Take notes in each interview, including the name of the candidate, the name and phone number of each reference, the date of the conversation, and answers to the following questions.

When did she work for you? For how long? How did you hire her? Why did she leave and with how much notice?

What were the gender and ages of the children when she started? What were her responsibilities with respect to the children, the household?

What was your overall impression of her? What did she do particularly well?

Is there anything you would change about her? What could she have done better? Did she have any limitations, physically or emotionally? Did her personal life ever interfere with her job? How did the two of you handle disagreements?

Describe her personality.

Would you say she demonstrates...

- Warmth and caring?
- Patience?
- Creativity?
- Initiative?
- A high energy level?
- A positive attitude?
- Promptness and reliability?
- Good judgment?
- Respect to the parents?

How did she deal with discipline issues? Did you ever suspect child abuse? Did you do a background check covering criminal, credit, driving, and child abuse?

How did she deal with emergencies? Please give me an example.

How healthy was she? Did you require her to have a physical and TB test?

Was there any evidence of drug or alcohol abuse? How often did she call in sick or unable to work?

How was her cleanliness? Her grooming?

How were her language skills? Could she write down messages? Read to the kids? Communicate with you easily? Did she keep a log of your child's day?

How often would she have visitors? Make or receive phone calls? Watch TV or just idle?

What was her schedule? Was she flexible if needed? Did she have other commitments?

Would you hire her again?

Would you be willing to share pay and benefit information?

What did you find was the best way to develop a good working relationship with her? Anything else I should know about her? Can I call you again if I have more questions?

NOTES

● ● ● CAREGIVER INTERVIEW

Conduct this interview in person so you can listen to the candidate's answers and observe her demeanor. Above, all, trust your instincts.

To begin, welcome the applicant. Tell her about your family and home. Review the positive things you've heard about her. Explain the interview process. Take notes during the interview, including the name and phone number of the candidate, the date of the interview, and answers to the following questions.

BACKGROUND

- Why do you wish to be a caregiver? What are your long-term goals?
- Tell me about your family and your interests. If you have children, who takes care of them? What about when they're sick?
- Where do you live? How long have you been there and do you plan to stay there?
- What is your education? Any special training in childcare? Are you certified in CPR/First Aid for infants? (If so, when and where were you certified?)

CHILDCARE EXPERIENCE

- How many families have you worked with? How many years of childcare experience do you have?
- For the last three jobs/families: Describe your employers and their children. (Make sure she addresses: duration of her job, ages of children, responsibilities, likes/dislikes, why she left, and pay/benefits.)

Tell me about your childhood.

What are your greatest strengths?

In what areas could you improve?

What do you think a baby's needs are from a caregiver? What is your role?

Give me an example of an emergency you had to deal with in taking care of children?

What would you do if a baby were choking? Unconscious? Hurt or bleeding?

How do you think a child should be disciplined? When would you spank or hit a child?

What gets you frustrated? What do you do when you get frustrated?

Imagine my baby hadn't stopped crying for one hour straight. You've tried everything and now you're getting fed up. What would you do? (Hint: Put baby down in safe place like crib and take a breather nearby.)

Imagine you're bathing my baby and the doorbell rings. I had told you I was expecting an important delivery. What would you do? (Hint: Never leave baby unattended in the bath.)

How do you feel about putting babies on a schedule for naps and meals?

What kinds of things would you do with my baby? What would a typical day be like?

Give me an example of a disagreement you had with a former employer and how it was resolved.

Are you a U.S. citizen? If not, what is your status?

How long have you been in the U.S.? Why did you leave your country of origin? How long do you expect to stay?

Do you have family outside this area? If so, do you need to visit them? How often and for how long?

- How comfortable are you with answering the phone and taking messages? Answering the door if I am expecting someone?
- Do you swim? Do you play any sports? Do you speak any foreign languages? Do you have any special skills?
- Do you have any pets? How comfortable are you with pets? Are you willing to help care for our pets?
- Do you smoke?
- Do you have any health issues? Any physical restrictions or allergies? How many sick days have you taken in the last few years?
- When was your most recent physical? Last TB test? Do you have health insurance?
- How would you get to and from work? If you drive, what happens if your car breaks down?
- How long have you had a driver's license? Any accidents? Speeding tickets? Do you have auto insurance?
- Have you ever been arrested or had any problems with the law?
- Will you agree to a criminal, driving, credit, social security (or work authorization) and child abuse background check?
- Will you agree to a physical, including a TB screening?
- Are you willing to take a CPR/First Aid class if I pay for it?

SCHEDULE

- When are you available weekdays and weekends? Do you have any constraints (jobs, family, school, church) weekdays or weekends?
- Are you available overnight? Are you willing to travel on vacations with us? Are you willing to take your vacation time while we're on vacation?
- Are you interviewing with other families right now? When would you be able to start?

RESPONSIBILITIES

- Review the Job Description, including pay and benefits. How does that sound?

◉ What do you need/expect from this job? What qualities are you looking for in a family?

◉ Do you need to receive phone calls? Visitors? Do you have special dietary needs?

CAREGIVER'S QUESTIONS

◉ Do you have any questions for me? Is there anything else you'd like to tell me about yourself?

TOUR/TIME WITH BABY

◉ Show her around your home. For live-in caregivers, show her living quarters. Introduce a viable candidate to your baby.

MY OBSERVATIONS

◉ Was she prompt for the interview? Does she seem competent and reliable? How was she with my baby? Did she light up when talking about other children she's cared for? Do her personality and her values mesh with our family? What did her body language tell me? How was her appearance, neat and clean? Can she communicate adequately? Am I comfortable with her? What's my gut feeling?

NOTES

NOTES

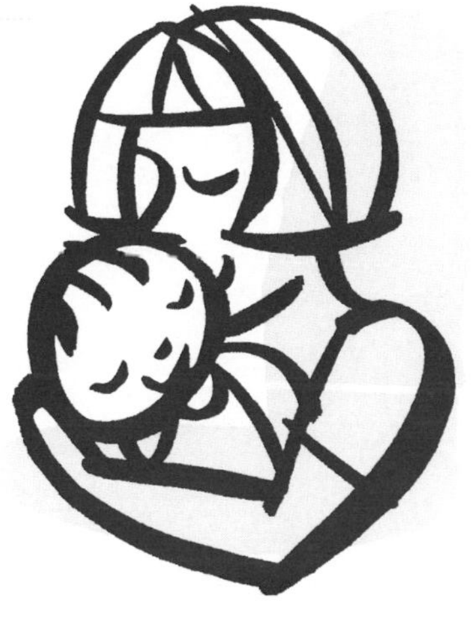

DAYCARE INTERVIEW AND TOUR

Nothing compares to an on-site visit of daycare facilities to help you make up your mind. Can you picture your child here? Do you feel comfortable in the environment and with the staff? Above all, listen to your gut feeling. Take notes in each interview, including the name and phone number of the daycare, the name of the person you interview, the date of the interview, and answers to the following questions.

BASICS AND PHILOSOPHY

- Is your daycare licensed and inspected? Accredited? How long have you been in business?
- What is the center's philosophy of care? What are its goals?
- How many children are enrolled in the center? What is the age range?
- Is there a separate room for infants with dedicated caregivers? What is the maximum number of babies in the infant room (ideally no more than 6)?
- Are children supervised at all times? What is your infant to staff ratio (ideally no more than 3 to 1)? Will the same person take care of my baby each day?
- How do caregivers stimulate infants throughout the day? How much time do infants spend in bouncer seats, swings, etc?
- What is a typical day like? Is there a schedule of activities? Is there time set aside for outside play? How much TV viewing do you allow?
- How do you respond to a crying baby? How do you discipline a child? How do you handle disruptive children (hitting, biting, etc.)?

FEEDING, SLEEPING, DIAPERING

- Are infants held when they are fed bottles? Will you give my baby my breast milk instead of formula? How will you store my milk?
- Are infants put on a schedule? Are there nap times? How are the parents' wishes taken into consideration?
- How often are baby diapers changed? Where? How do you keep track? How are diapers disposed of?

- How, and how often, do you communicate with parents regarding their child's behavior, progress, and needs as well as daycare news? (e.g. open houses, newsletters, conferences.)
- Do the child's primary caregivers maintain a written log book with daily entries? Can parents review it at their discretion?
- Is parent participation encouraged? Can I visit at any time without notice?

HEALTH ISSUES

- What is your policy regarding sick babies? How often does the center experience outbreaks of serious illness? How are parents notified of outbreaks? How would we be notified if there were an illness or injury involving our baby?
- How does the center handle children with allergies or special needs? Will the staff administer medications prescribed for my baby? How do you keep track?
- Are medical records clearly posted for each child? Is emergency information in plain view? Where are medications stored?

STAFF/TRAINING

- What do you look for when interviewing candidates for staff positions?
- What is the educational background of the staff? Any training in early childhood education or child development?
- Is the staff CPR and First Aid certified for infants? How often is their certification renewed?
- Are federal background checks done on all employees, including criminal and child abuse checks? Are all employees required to pass regular physical exams and to be up-to-date on all immunizations?
- What staff turnover do you experience? How long have staff members been with the center, on average? Will you notify us if and when a new caregiver is assigned to our baby?

- What safety measures do you have in place? How are the doors secured?
- Are smoke detectors present? Where are the fire exits? Are fire drills conducted monthly?
- Are cleaning products, medicine and other toxic substances locked up at all times?
- How old are the cribs and other equipment? How often are linens changed? Does each infant have his/her own crib?
- How old are the toys? How often are they cleaned and replaced?
- How do you keep up with product recalls?
- When is the staff required to wash their hands? To wash the children's hands?
- What is the policy for having someone else pick up my child?

- What are your center's hours and holiday schedule?
- Will you accommodate early drop-offs or late pick-ups? Is there a fee?
- What are your fees? Do they change for older children? How often are they raised? Are there additional fees? Will you charge us when we're on vacation or when our child is ill at home?
- What do I need to provide for my child? All bottles and snacks? Diapers and other supplies?
- How do I sign up? Is there a waiting list?
- How is separation between the child and parents handled? How long can parents remain at the daycare for transition purposes?
- May I have three references of parents who have their babies enrolled with you?

- How close is the center to my home? My work?
- Are there age-appropriate toys and activities, indoors and out?

- Is the center safe and sanitary? Organized and clutter-free? Bright and well lit? Check the food preparation, sleeping, and eating areas, as well as bathrooms.
- Is the center childproofed? Are there safety issues like cords or tipping hazards? Is the outside area fenced in and removed from nearby streets?
- Is emergency information posted clearly? Phone numbers for fire, police, ambulance, poison control? Where are first aid items kept?
- Are all children under constant and attentive supervision?
- What are caregivers doing with infants? Do they hold them, talk and sing to them? When I ask them about each child, do they seem to know the child, his/her needs and personality?
- Does each baby have a crib and cubby space personalized with his own toys, pacifiers and pictures?
- Do the children's charts seem complete, up-to-date, filled with thoughtful and detailed entries?
- Do the children and caregivers seem happy and active? Is the general mood one of joyful play?
- Are the director and infant-room staff genuinely interested in my baby and eager to answer my questions and concerns?

NOTES

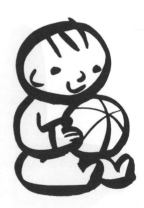

● ● ● BOOKS FOR MOM AND DAD

PREGNANCY AND DELIVERY

Brasner, Shari E., M.D. *Advice from a Pregnant Obstetrician: An Insider's Guide.* New York: Hyperion, 1998.

Curtis, Glade B., M.D. *Your Pregnancy Week by Week,* 4th ed. Tucson, AZ: Fisher Books, 2000.

Eisenberg, Arlene, Heidi E. Murkoff, and Sandee E. Hathaway. *What to Expect When You're Expecting,* 2d ed. New York: Workman, 1996.

Harris, A. Christine. *The Pregnancy Journal: A Day-to-Day Guide to a Healthy and Happy Pregnancy.* San Francisco: Chronicle Books, 1996.

Iovine, Vicki. *The Girlfriends' Guide to Pregnancy: Or Everything Your Doctor Won't Tell You.* New York: Pocket Books, 1995.

PRENATAL NUTRITION AND EXERCISE

Clapp, James F. III, M.D. *Exercising through Your Pregnancy.* Champaign, IL: Human Kinetics, 1998.

Fitness Magazine with Ginny Graves. *Pregnancy Fitness.* New York: Crown Publishing Group, 1999.

Swinney, Bridget, with Tracy Anderson. *Eating Expectantly: A Practical and Tasty Approach to Prenatal Nutrition.* Minnetonka, MN: Meadowbrook Press, 2000.

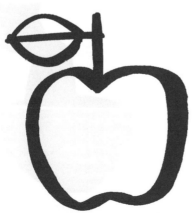

Lansky, Bruce. *Baby Names around the World.* Minnetonka, MN: Meadowbrook Press, 1999.

Rosenkranz, Linda, and Pamela Redmond Satran. *Beyond Jennifer and Jason, Madison and Montana: What to Name Your Baby Now.* New York: St. Martin's Griffin, 1999.

Rosenkranz, Linda, and Pamela Redmond Satran. *The Last Word on First Names: The Definitive A–Z Guide to the Best and Worst in Baby Names by America's Leading Experts.* New York: St. Martin's Press, 1995.

Satran, Pamela Redmond, and Linda Rosenkranz. *The Baby Naming Journal.* San Francisco: Chronicle Books, 2000.

Brazelton, T. Berry, M.D. *Touchpoints: Your Child's Emotional and Behavioral Development.* Reading, MA: Addison-Wesley, 1994.

Eisenberg, Arlene, Heidi E. Murkoff, and Sandee E. Hathaway. *What to Expect the First Year.* New York: Workman, 1989.

Fries, James F., M.D., and Donald M. Vickery, M.D. *Taking Care of Your Child: A Parent's Illustrated Guide to Complete Medical Care,* 5th ed. Reading, MA: Perseus Books, 1999.

Greenspan, Stanley I., M.D., with Nancy Breslau Lewis. *Building Healthy Minds: The Six Experiences that Create Intelligence and Emotional Growth in Babies and Young Children.* Cambridge, MA: Perseus Books, 1999.

Leach, Penelope. *Your Baby and Child: From Birth to Age Five,* 3d ed. New York: Alfred A. Knopf, 1997.

Sears, William, M.D., and Martha Sears. *The Baby Book: Everything You Need to Know about Your Baby—From Birth to Age Two.* Boston: Little, Brown, 1993.

Shelov, Steven P., M.D., and Robert E. Hannemann, M.D., eds. *The American Academy of Pediatrics Caring for Your Baby and Young Child: Birth to Age 5,* rev. ed. New York: Bantam Books, 1998.

Spock, Benjamin, M.D., and Steven J. Parker, M.D. *Dr. Spock's Baby and Child Care*, *7th ed.* New York: Pocket Books, 1998.

Tamborlane, William V., M.D., ed. *The Yale Guide to Children's Nutrition.* New Haven, CT: Yale University Press, 1997.

NURSING

Eiger, Marvin S., M.D., and Sally Wendkos Olds. *The Complete Book of Breastfeeding*, 3rd ed. New York: Workman, 1999.

Huggins, Kathleen. *The Nursing Mother's Companion*, 4th ed. Boston, MA: Harvard Common Press, 1999.

Torgus, Judy, and Gwen Gotsch, eds. *La Leche League International The Womanly Art of Breastfeeding*, 6th ed. Schaumburg, IL: La Leche League International, 1997.

BABY SOOTHING AND SLEEP

Ferber, Richard, M.D., *Solve Your Child's Sleep Problems.* New York: Simon and Schuster, 1985.

Sammons, William A. H., M.D., *The Self-Calmed Baby: A Liberating New Approach to Parenting Your Infant.* Boston: Little, Brown, 1989.

Weissbluth, Marc, M.D., *Healthy Sleep Habits, Happy Child*, rev. ed. New York: Ballantine, 1999.

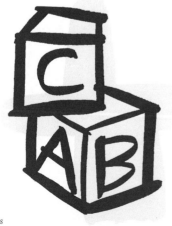

Acredolo, Linda, and Susan Goodwyn. *Baby Signs: How to Talk with Your Baby Before Your Baby Can Talk.* Chicago, IL: Contemporary Books, 1996.

Lansky, Vicki. *Games Babies Play: From Birth to Twelve Months.* New York: MJF Books, 1998.

Moore, Jack. *97 Ways to Make a Baby Laugh.* New York: Workman, 1997.

Warner, Penny. *Baby Play and Learn.* Minnetonka, MN: Meadowbrook Press, 1999.

Agnew, Connie L., M.D., Alan H. Klein, M.D., and Jill Alison Ganon. *Twins! Expert Advice from Two Practicing Physicians on Pregnancy, Birth, and the First Year of Life with Twins.* New York: Harper Collins, 1997.

Malmstrom, Patricia Maxwell, and Janet Poland. *The Art of Parenting Twins: The Unique Joys and Challenges of Raising Twins and Other Multiples.* New York: Ballantine, 1999.

Tinglof, Christina Baglivi. *Double Duty: The Parent's Guide to Raising Twins from Pregnancy through the School Years.* Lincolnwood, IL: Contemporary Books, 1998.

Gotsch, Gwen. *La Leche League International Breastfeeding Your Premature Baby,* rev ed. Schaumburg, IL: La Leche League International, 1999.

Linden, Dana Wechsler, Emma Trenti Paroli, and Mia Wechsler Doron, M.D., *Preemies: The Essential Guide for Parents of Premature Babies.* New York: Pocket Books, 2000.

Tracy, Amy E., and Dianne I. Maroney. *Your Premature Baby and Child: Helpful Answers and Advice for Parents.* New York: Berkley, 1999.

Barrett, Nina. *I Wish Someone Had Told Me: A Realistic Guide to Early Motherhood.* Chicago: Academy Chicago Publishers, 1997.

Bing, Elizabeth, and Libby Colman. *Laughter and Tears: The Emotional Life of New Mothers.* New York: H. Holt, 1997.

Iovine, Vicki. *The Girlfriend's Guide to Surviving the First Year of Motherhood: Wise and Witty Advice on Everything from Coping with Postpartum Mood Swings to Salvaging Your Sex Life to Fitting into That Favorite Pair of Jeans.* New York: Berkley, 1997.

Lamott, Anne. *Operating Instructions: A Journal of My Son's First Year.* New York: Pantheon Books, 1993.

FATHERS

Barron, James Douglas. *She's Had a Baby—and I'm Having a Meltdown: What Every New Father Needs to Know about Marriage, Sex, and Diapers.* New York: Quill, 1999.

Frank, Robert, with Kathryn E. Livingston. *The Involved Father: Family-Tested Solutions for Getting Dads to Participate More in the Daily Lives of Their Children.* New York: St. Martin's Press, 1999.

Nelson, Kevin. *The Daddy Guide: Real-Life Advice and Tips from over 250 Dads and Other Experts.* Lincolnwood, IL: Contemporary Books, 1998.

PARENTING

Cline, Foster, M.D., and Jim Fay. *Parenting with Love and Logic: Teaching Children Responsibility.* Colorado Springs, CO: Navpress, 1990.

Eyre, Linda and Richard. *Three Steps to a Strong Family.* New York: Simon and Schuster, 1994.

Jordan, Pamela L., Scott M. Stanley, and Howard J. Markman. *Becoming Parents: How to Strengthen Your Marriage as Your Family Grows.* San Francisco: Jossey-Bass Pub., 1999.

Sanders, Darcie, and Martha M. Bullen. *Staying Home: From Full-Time Professional to Full-Time Parent.* Boston, Little, Brown, 1992.

Vannoy, Steven W. *The 10 Greatest Gifts I Give My Children: Parenting from the Heart.* New York, Simon and Schuster, 1994.

CHILDCARE

Carlton, Susan, and Coco Myers. *The Nanny Book: The Smart Parent's Guide to Hiring, Firing, and Every Sticky Situation in between.* New York: St.

Martin's Griffin, 1999.

Ehrich, Michelle. *The Anxious Parent's Guide to Quality Childcare: An Informative, Step-by-Step Manual on Finding and Keeping the Finest Care for Your Child.* New York: Berkley, 1999.

Porrazzo, Kimberly A. *The Nanny Kit: Everything You Need to Hire the Right Nanny.* New York: Penguin Books, 1999.

Sagel, Gail, and Lori Berke. *Making Childcare Choices: How to Find, Hire, and Keep the Best Childcare for Your Kids.* Holbrook, MA: Adams Media, 1999.

PRODUCT INFORMATION

Fields, Denise and Alan. Baby Bargains. *Secrets to Saving 20% to 50% on Baby Furniture, Equipment, Clothes, Toys, Maternity Wear and Much, Much More!* 3rd ed. Boulder, CO: Windsor Peak Press, 1999.

Lipper, Ari and Joanna. *Baby Stuff: A No-Nonsense Shopping Guide for Every Parent's Lifestyle.* New York: Dell Trade Paperback, 1997.

Oppenheim, Joanne and Stephanie. *Oppenheim Toy Portfolio 2000 Edition: The Best Toys, Books, Videos, Music and Software for Kids.* New York: Oppenheim Toy Portfolio, 1999.

Oppenheim, Joanne and Stephanie. *Oppenheim Toy Portfolio Baby and Toddler Play Book: From Patty-Cake to Teddy Bears—Everything You Need to Know about Playing with Your Baby and Toddler.* New York: Oppenheim Toy Portfolio, 1999.

Yager, Cary O. *Unbelievably Good Deals That You Absolutely Can't Get Unless You're a Parent,* rev. ed. Lincolnwood, IL: Contemporary, 2000.

SAFETY

Brandenburg, Mark A., M.D., *Child Safe: A Practical Guide for Preventing Childhood Injuries.* New York: Three Rivers Press, 2000.

Stone, Leslie, Larry Stone, and Laurie Levy. *The Safe and Sound Child.* Glenview, IL: GoodYearBooks, 1996.

Wolf, Cindy. *On the Safe Side: Your Complete Reference to Childproofing for Infants and Toddlers.* Wichita, KS: Whirlwind Pub, 1998.

MISCELLANEOUS

Berman, Eleanor. *Grandparenting ABC's: A Beginner's Handbook.* New York: Berkley, 1998.

Johnson, Sue, and Julie Carlson. *Grandloving: Making Memories with Your Grandchildren,* 2d ed. Fairport, NY: Heartstrings Press, 2000.

Keliman, Karen, and Valerie D. Raskin, M.D., *This Isn't What I Expected: Overcoming Postpartum Depression.* New York: Bantam Books, 1994.

Kelsh, Nick. *How to Photograph Your Baby: Getting Close, with Your Camera and Your Heart.* New York: Smithmark, 1999.

● ● ● **MAGAZINES**

American Baby: 800-678-1208 (free)
Baby Talk/Healthy Pregnancy: 800-264-9871
Child: 800-777-0222
Fit Pregnancy: 800-967-2084
Parenting: 800-264-9871
Parents: 800-727-3682
Twins: 888-55TWINS
Working Mother: 800-627-0690

● ● ● **CATALOGS/MAIL ORDER**

MATERNITY AND NURSING

Athleta: 888-322-5515; athleta.com
Belly Basics: 800-496-6684; bellybasics.com
Bravado Designs: 800-590-7802; bravadodesigns.com
Garnet Hill: 800-622-6216; garnethill.com
Japanese Weekend: 800-808-0555; japaneseweekend.com
JC Penney Maternity: 800-222-6161; jcpenney.com
La Leche League: 800-LALECHE; lalecheleague.org
L'Attesa: 800-327-2040; lattesa.com
Liz Lange Maternity: 888-616-5777; lizlange.com
Mama Bella: 888-FIT-MAMA; mamabella.com

Motherwear: 800-950-2500; motherwear.com

Nurturing Mother's Boutique: 888-MOMSBAGS; momsbags.com

Pumpkin Maternity: 877-460-0337; pumpkinmaternity.com

BABY CLOTHING AND GEAR

Baby Catalog of America: 800-PLAYPEN; babycatalog.com

Biobottoms: 800-766-1254; biobottoms.com

The Company Store: 800-356-9367; thecompanystore.com

Garnet Hill: 800-622-6216; garnethill.com

Hanna Andersson: 800-222-0544; hannaandersson.com

JC Penney: 800-222-6161; jcpenney.com

The Land of Nod: 800-933-9904; thelandofnod.com

Land's End: 800-356-4444; landsend.com

LL Bean: 800-221-4221; llbean.com

One Step Ahead: 800-274-8440; onestepahead.com

Pottery Barn Kids: 800-430-7373; potterybarn.com

The Right Start: 800-LITTLE1; rightstart.com

Talbot's Kids: 800-TALBOTS; talbots.com

SAFETY

Perfectly Safe: 800-837-KIDS; kidsstuff.com

Safe Beginnings: 800-598-8911; safebeginnings.com

Safety 1st: 800-723-3065; safety1st.com

ANNOUNCEMENTS AND ALBUMS

Artitudes (adoption): 800-741-0711; miracleofadoption.com

Exposures: 800-222-4947; exposuresonline.com

H&F Announcements: 800-964-4002; hfproducts.com

TOYS, BOOKS, AND MUSIC

Chinaberry: 800-776-2242, chinaberry.com

Constructive Playthings: 800-832-0572, constplay.com

FAO Schwarz: 800-426-TOYS, faoschwarz.com

Fisher Price: 800-432-5437, fisherprice.com

Imagine The Challenge: 888-777-1493; imaginetoys.com

Lilly's Kids: 800-LILLIAN, lillianvernon.com

Music for Little People: 800-409-2457, mflp.com

Sensational Beginnings: 800-444-2147, sensationalbeginnings.com

The Walt Disney Catalog: 800-237-5751, disneystore.com

● ◦ ● **WEB SITES**

PREGNANCY AND PARENTING

babycenter.com

babyzone.com

bosombuddies.com (nursing)

childbirth.org

family.com

iparenting.com

networkingmoms.com (working moms)

parenting-qa.com

parentsoup.com

parentsplace.com

preemieparents.com

slowlane.com (stay-at-home Dads)

storksite.com

twinstuff.com

HEALTH AND SAFETY

childrecall.com

medscape.com

pedsnet.org

safebaby.net

CHILDCARE

4nannies.com

carefinder.com

edaycare.com

nannynetwork.com

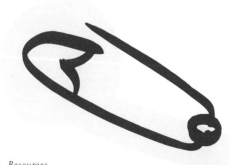

ORGANIZATIONS, ASSOCIATIONS, AGENCIES, SERVICES

PREGNANCY AND CHILDBIRTH

American Academy of Husband Coached Childbirth (Bradley method): 800-423-2397; bradleybirth.com

American College of Nurse-Midwives: 888-MIDWIFE; midwife.org

Association of Labor Assistants and Childbirth Educators: 888-222-5223; alace.org

Doulas of North America: 801-756-7331; dona.com

Lamaze International: 800-368-4404; Lamaze-childbirth.com

Midwives Alliance of North America: 888-923-MANA; mana.org

Sidelines (high risk pregnancies, bed rest): 949-497-2265; sidelines.org

HEALTHCARE

American Academy of Pediatrics: 847-228-5005; aap.org

American College of Obstetricians and Gynecologists: 800-762-2264; acog.org

National Immunization Program: 800-232-2522; cdc.gov/nip

SIDS Alliance: 800-221-7437; sidsalliance.org

PARENTING

Single Parents Association: 800-704-2102

US Labor Dept. Family Leave Hotline: 800-959-FMLA

SPECIAL INTEREST MOM

Depression After Delivery: 800-944-4773; behavenet.com/dadinc

Mothers and More: 800-223-9399; femalehome.org

La Leche League (nursing): 800-LALECHE; lalecheleague.org

Mothers of Supertwins: 631-859-1110; mostonline.org

National Domestic Violence Hotline: 800-799-7233; ndvh.org

National Organization of Mothers of Twins Club: 877-540-2200; nomotc.org

National Organization of Single Mothers: 704-888-KIDS; singlemothers.org

Postpartum Support International: 805-967-7636; postpartum.net

American Association of Poison Control Centers: aapcc.org

Auto Safety Hotline (car seat safety): 888-DASH-2-DOT; nhtsa.org

Baby's Away (baby supplies rental): 800-571-0077; babysaway.com

Babywatch (nanny surveillance): 800-558-5669; babywatch.com

Juvenile Products Manufacturers Association: jpma.org

National Association of Diaper Services: 610-971-4850; diapernet.com

Child Help USA (national child abuse hotline): 800-422-4453; childhelpusa.org

National Safe Kids Campaign (car seat safety): 800-441-1888; safekids.org

US Consumer Product Safety Commission (product recalls): 800-638-CPSC; cpsc.gov

AuPairCare: 800-4-AUPAIR; aupaircare.com

Childcare Aware: 800-424-2246; childcareaware.org

EF Au Pair: 800-333-6056; efaupair.com

Internal Revenue Service: 800-829-1040; irs.gov

International Au Pair Association: iapa.org

International Nanny Association: 800-297-1477; nanny.org

Nanny Tax, Inc.: 212-867-1776; nannytax.com

National Association for Family Child Care: 800-359-3817; nafcc.org

National Association for the Education of Young Children: 800-424-2460; naeyc.org

National Child Care Information Center: 800-616-2242; nccic.org

National Resource Center for Health and Safety in Childcare: 800-598-KIDS

On-Line Screening Services, Inc. (background checks): 800-358-5383; onlinescreening.com

● ● ● NOTES

● ○ ● **NOTES**